What people are saying about

Breath for Health

In my travels around the yoga world investigating the teaching of different traditions, the breath work taught by students of Krishnamacharya in his later life was the most subtle and profound I encountered. *Breath for Health* presents a program based on these principles that allows even raw beginners to learn the basics of healthy breathing, and then step-by-step safely build up to more advanced practices. The results for health and well-being following this deceptively simple program can be life-changing.

Dr Timothy McCall, author of *Yoga as Medicine: The Yogic Prescription for Health and Healing*, co-editor and contributor, *The Principles and Practice of Yoga in Health Care*

A reading of this book makes it clear that Michael has taken all precautions to present the lessons in a very simple but accurate way. Interspersed with a lot of technical points and references to medical science, the step-by-step method adds value for lay practitioners. I congratulate Michael on his attempt to make the complex science of Prāṇāyāma simple, in which he has succeeded.

Yogācārya S Sridharan, advisor, senior mentor, Yoga Therapist Krishnamacharya Yoga Mandiram, Chennai and Member of the Governing Council of the MDNIY (India's Morarji Desai National Institute of Yoga)

Breathing is multi-dimensional, and when taught by the right teacher, it has the power to transform physical and mental health for the better. These tools should be accessible to everyone and *Breath for Health* offers the gateway to just that.

Patrick McKeown, author of *The Oxygen Advantage*, *Atomic Focus* and *The Breathing Cure*

Michael Hutchinson has written the guide to breathing that every yoga practitioner, yoga teacher and yoga therapist needs to have on their bookshelf. This is a guide to learning and teaching breathwork that lays out simple practices for everybody, yet offers tremendous depth and subtlety. I will be using this book for all of my yoga and yoga therapy trainings going forward.

Dr Amy Wheeler, Ph.D & C-IAYT, former president of the Board of the International Association of Yoga Therapists (2018–2020)

Currently, most articles and books dealing with yoga are either oriented towards postures (āsana) or towards the philosophy of yoga. Few books deal with breathing. This is why Michael's fills me with joy. This is a useful and quality work; I wish him great success and thank him for this contribution.

Frans Moors, co-author of *The Viniyoga of Yoga*, and personal student of TKV Desikachar

Breath is essential to life, and how we breathe affects the quality of our health and well-being. Michael's book is a guide to harnessing these qualities. Yoga's wisdom has inspired his approach and links us to the understanding that breath is life.

Gillian Lloyd, personal student of TKV Desikachar, former chair of Viniyoga Britain

Breath for Health

A Mindful Way to Restore Your Natural
Breathing Cycle

Breath for Health

A Mindful Way to Restore Your Natural
Breathing Cycle

Michael Hutchinson

BOOKS

Winchester, UK
Washington, USA

JOHN HUNT PUBLISHING

First published by O-Books, 2023
O-Books is an imprint of John Hunt Publishing Ltd., 3 East St., Alresford,
Hampshire SO24 9EE, UK
office@jhpbooks.com
www.johnhuntpublishing.com
www.o-books.com

For distributor details and how to order please visit the 'Ordering' section on our website.

Text copyright: Michael Hutchinson 2022

ISBN: 978 1 80341 440 9
978 1 80341 441 6 (ebook)
Library of Congress Control Number: 2022949215

A CIP catalogue record for this book is available from the British Library.

Design: Lapiz Digital Services

UK: Printed and bound by CPI Group (UK) Ltd, Croydon, CR0 4YY
Printed in North America by CPI GPS partners

The author of this book does not dispense medical advice or prescribe the use of any technique as a form of treatment for physical, emotional, or medical problems without the advice of a physician, either directly or indirectly. The intent of the author is only to offer information of a general nature to help you in your quest for emotional and spiritual well-being. In the event you use any of the information in this book for yourself, which is your constitutional right, the author and the publisher assume no responsibility for your actions.

We operate a distinctive and ethical publishing philosophy in all areas of our business, from our global network of authors to production and worldwide distribution.

Contents

Dedication

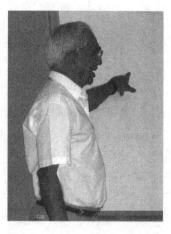

This book is dedicated to the memory of our great teacher, Srī TKV Desikachar, who continues to point the way for us all.

Forewords

Our breath, essential and all pervading, yet so often mysterious, is explored simply and lightly in this delightful book.

Michael, scientist and long-term yoga practitioner, makes the case that throughout human evolution our body has adapted to breathe optimally in a particular way. Yet changing lifestyles and challenges often create a disconnection from healthy breathing patterns.

Presented in such brevity, we learn how optimal breathing was observed and practised by the ancient yogis who also sought the best health. Michael has looked to current scientific models as well as ancient teachings and past teachers for guidance. In this book, we can see the synergy of these two factors at work, well researched and clear, presenting links which otherwise may have remained unconnected or out of reach, and with acute relevance in this present moment.

The addition of pictures illustrating breathing practices provides a step-by-step method and support for putting research and recommendations into action. The underpinning reference to the work of Krishnamacharya and TKV Desikachar brings their potentially life-changing work to the mainstream, a real achievement.

This great task has been accomplished in a way that is simple and light for a beginner, yet still educational and thought provoking for the more experienced. In sharing his work, Michael provides a valuable wealth of knowledge delivered with his usual gentle humility.

Maggie Shanks, vice-chair, Society of Yoga Practitioners, March 2022

Breath for Health is a clear and concise book that is invaluable to anyone who desires to know more about breathing and how different techniques can shift the state of our body and mind. There is elegance in simplicity and Michael has successfully written a book that is understandable to beginners, but also has depth for more advanced practitioners. Breath and breathing are the essence of all yoga practices. Without understanding the breath, we cannot understand yoga. For any reader who would like to learn authentic yoga in the tradition of TKV Desikachar from South India, author of *The Heart of Yoga*, this book is a requirement for their studies.

Although written to appeal to everyone, *Breath for Health* is also a book that avid students of yoga will find fascinating, that yoga teachers and therapists need to receive more clarity for their teaching, and that healthcare providers can use to understand the importance of breathing properly for health and healing. While most people, including teachers and healthcare providers, now understand the importance of mindfulness, what they may not understand is that there is a pre-requisite for inner moments of stillness to occur. Michael has coined the term 'Breathfulness.' That is to say that where the breath goes, the mind follows. When our breathing is erratic and inconsistent, in response to the stresses of our lives, we lose connection with the deeper parts of ourselves. Hence, there is no mindfulness of the inner landscape without first having self-connection to our breath.

I think that Michael is the perfect person to bring these ancient teachings forward. He is a yoga practitioner and scientist who has practiced these techniques daily for nearly 40 years. He has studied deeply for decades in the tradition of T. Krishnamacharya and TKV Desikachar. We need more of these balanced people writing books; people who appreciate physiology and anatomy as well as the mystery of the human system and flow of what the rishis called prana, or life-force. Michael's goal was to keep this book simple, elegant and easy to apply. He has outlined many breathing exercises so that we can experience the techniques. He tells stories and then backs up the techniques with scientific explanations of what is happening both in the anatomy and physiology. Michael's text is supported by Mandy Meaden's clear images that make it easy to understand what is happening during the different phases of the breath and beyond.

My favorite part of the book is the discussions on breath and the relationship to posture, how to build appropriate ratios and the intricacies of nostril regulation for different effects on body and mind. I know that you will enjoy this book and I hope that if you are a yoga teacher or yoga therapist, you will consider using it in your trainings. This is the book that my students have desired for decades. Thank goodness that Michael has taken the time to write the ancient teachings down with precision and clarity.

Amy Wheeler, former president of the Board of the International Association of Yoga Therapists, October 2022

Preface

Well before the recent pandemic, I'd written a synopsis for a small workbook on 'befriending the breath'. Also, for a couple of years, I'd been running some 'Breath 4 Health' classes at a local community centre. However, starting in March 2020, there was so much disruption and we were all suffering to a lesser or greater extent; my aim was to contribute what I could by means of online teaching of breathwork. Out of these Zoom classes arose, by January 2021, the first draft of this book.

In 2020-21, I could only reach a few dozen people. I hope this book will reach out to far more of you who are interested in breathing. That could be for your health, physical or mental, or to enhance your meditation practice, or because you are yourself a teacher or exercise therapist, seeking to help people through instructing them in breathing.

More recently, I've been able to follow some leads, especially into respiratory physiology, and have found research that underpins the breathwork we were taught by Desikachar.

Some of you may bear the scars of this pandemic in the form of deep personal losses or a long-term setback to your health. These experiences may have made you very nervous about doing any work with your breath – breath is precious. However, a little volume that can be dipped into privately may be your way of beginning again. If only this book could have been put into my hands years ago, when I was a tense, introspective teenager; how much difference it would have made!

By way of acknowledgements, I'd like to start by thanking Paul Harvey, who was the mentor and tutor responsible for supporting my early development as a yoga therapist. Through Paul and a Tantric teacher, Muz Murray, I met my future mentor and guide, Gill Lloyd, who continues to give me encouragement and support. Gill also put me in touch with my illustrator,

4

Mandy Meaden, whose sensitive drawings add a lot to this volume.

I must also thank my dear wife, Linda, for her patience and support during the time I've been writing this book and her kind editing of this final version. Others who've helped with comments and encouragement on earlier drafts include fellow yoga teachers Jane Reynolds, Marian Thornley, Christina Jones, Maggie Shanks, Annemarie Visser and, for a medical opinion, Dr Martin Haslam.

Inspired by other writers and researchers in the field of breathwork, whom I've acknowledged at appropriate points, I have discovered further scientific backing for the breathing practices which Mr Desikachar learnt from his father and taught to us, based on centuries of tradition and experience.

No acknowledgement would be complete without thanking my students; I'm sorry there's not space to mention you all. If you are reading this, just let me say that, when you share with me the difficulties you encounter, it's then that I am pressed into finding solutions. These answers to your problems have comprised a large part of this book.

Michael Hutchinson, September 2022

Introduction

Why read this book?

In a leaflet for patients, the University Hospital Southampton NHS Foundation Trust (2019) stated that: 'Approximately 6-12% of the population experience chronic breathing pattern disorders, but some people are more affected than others. Chronic (long-term) changes in your breathing pattern can be very subtle and may happen over a long period of time.'

Based on these percentages, we have, in the UK alone, millions of people who could be helped to better health through breathing exercises. And there may be those of us whose breathing patterns, while not sufficiently dysfunctional to come to the attention of the medical profession, may not be consistent with optimum health.

In 1988, I heard Dr Claude Lum interviewed on BBC Radio. He had developed a reputation among his colleagues at Papworth Hospital, Cambridge, UK for helping patients with inexplicable symptoms. He helped these patients by giving them simple breathing exercises, ones which were basic compared to many that are in this book.

You may already be aware that you could be breathing in a better way. Or you are curious to know if there might be gains to be made by improving your breathing. If so, this book can certainly help you. Major physical issues aside, all of us have the potential for optimal breathing; it's what we started out with in life; however, there are so many issues you must have encountered between early childhood and adult life that it's likely one or more of these will have affected your breathing pattern significantly. Working through the exercises in this book, taking just 10 minutes every day, you will gradually restore that fully functional breathing with which you began life.

I can promise this thanks to my unique background. While working as a scientist, but taking an interest in yoga for the sake of my health, I stumbled across a school of yoga with a unique focus on working with the breath. Realising the value of this for myself and others, I went on to train as a yoga therapist within this tradition. My experience gained from teaching others and my determination to optimise my own breathing, together with my capacity for scientific understanding of the role of the breath, has given me the knowledge and motivation to write this book – for you.

Once you have worked through this book, in your own time, you will feel fitter and better in yourself. If you're reading this as an adult, the aspect of yoga that will help you most with your responsibilities is the yoga of breathing; however, you can start working with this book as soon as you're in your teens. No standard of fitness is needed for you to start and, even if you consider yourself to be very fit, it's still likely that you have things to learn which will help you improve even further. You and your breath are going to be recruiting muscles you almost certainly haven't heard of and doing things you wouldn't have imagined.

The personal stories you will read at relevant points in this book will show you how my students have benefitted in ways that range from reduced or eliminated asthma symptoms to the capacity to lift greater weights without pain, all from focusing on their breathing. The breathing I taught someone disabled by a baffling illness brought a ray of light and hope into her very limited life.

So why put this off? Your breath is waiting to help you and working from this book for 10 minutes every day will show it how. A new era is coming where we, as patients, are going to be helping to plan our own healthcare goals. Why not make better breathing your first objective?

Background

The breathwork that I've been teaching for nearly 40 years has its roots in a centuries-old tradition whose revival began in the 1920s, at Mysore in India. The teacher, Professor T Krishnamacharya, often referred to as 'The father of modern Yoga', is known to the world mainly through his students, including BKS Iyengar. From the 1960s onwards, by then assisted by his son, TKV Desikachar, he adapted and combined bodily movements with these ancient breathwork methods to improve people's health and mobility.

What Mr Desikachar taught us, I've recently discovered, is in accordance with modern research into 'quiet', relaxed breathing, especially research initiated in the 1980s by Professor André de Troyer at the Brussels School of Medicine.

These remedial breathing methods developed by Mr Desikachar and his father have been taught to many tens of thousands of people in India and elsewhere. Using these same methods, I shall be leading you, step-by-step, towards recovering and reinforcing your natural breathing cycle, with positive consequences for your health and confidence. While there is no absolute right way to breathe for everyone in every situation, there is such a thing as an optimal breathing cycle, from when your breath starts to flow in until it finishes flowing out.

Although a scientist, accomplished in my own field, I'm not going to describe in detail the drawbacks, even dangers, of having acquired, through life, a sub-optimal habit of breathing. Instead, I shall focus on the positive, what you and your breath can do together, in partnership, to bring it around into better habits.

I'm sure there'll be some pleasant surprises for you on your journey through these exercises, as there have been for many of my students. As Mr Desikachar taught us, discovering your own potential is the most powerful way of learning.

Before you start

There is no pressure and, rather than rushing to try all the exercises at once, please work with each one in turn for a few days at least, before moving on to the next. In fact, so long as you are keeping up your practice almost every day for about 10 minutes, you can take as long as you need to get comfortable and feel practised with each exercise before moving on.

You are not going to fight any bad habits, but develop new and better ones. If you work steadily and patiently, you will make progress. Help and reassurance from someone experienced in practising and teaching breathwork in this way (see links in Chapter 8) can be invaluable, but please don't delay; this book will certainly get you started.

You won't need a lot of equipment. A yoga mat will be handy for some of the later exercises, also some foam yoga blocks (I suggest one thick and two thin), an upright chair and one or two cushions. To start, you'll need very little, but what you will need is to be mindful during the exercises and open to feeling how they are affecting you in one way or another.

These are not exercises which can be done mechanically while your attention is elsewhere. Please, let yourself be mindful and open to feeling what your breath is doing. No music, no phone, ten minutes of complete break. I'm hoping there will be some exercises that you actually find enjoyable as well as beneficial. These exercises can be kept up for as long as you like, while continuing to explore in this book.

As I suggested above, you may enjoy unexpected benefits; for example, one of my students reported that:

Compared to 10 years ago, when I was 21, I did a 10k run again this year (2021) and had an easier time thru utilizing breathing techniques/being mindful.
Jillian

Finally, please do not burden yourself with expectations of making rapid progress. That was a big mistake that I made when starting with yoga over 40 years ago; and please don't expect any straightforward, linear progress. By working patiently through this book, you will improve your breathing. There will, however, be times when you feel you've fallen back. Yet, once you realise what has happened and apply yourself again, you will improve further than before. Please relax and let the joy of free breathing take you over.

Advice

Nothing in these pages is intended to replace any medical treatment you may be either receiving or in need of. Although you personally may find certain exercises the most helpful for your condition and choose to practise them daily, no specific remedies are offered. Everyone's response to an exercise is individual, and this is particularly true of exercises with your breath.

Chapter 1

Breathing Is Not a 'Lost Art'

Every creature on this earth has to breathe, in one sense or another. Plants take in carbon dioxide and exhale oxygen. For us, and for other animals, it's the opposite. Nothing can live in a vacuum, sealed off from its environment. Yet we humans are unique in one way; we can control our breathing in more ways than any other creature. Part of the reason may lie with our distant ancestors, when they learnt to control fire. If you have ever pursed your lips and blown a long, smooth, steady breath onto some kindling, you can appreciate how this ability enabled our distant ancestors to keep warm, cook food and ward off predators.

EXERCISE 1.1: Blowing into the palm of your hand. Let's try this now. Take in a smooth, deep breath, through your nose if you can, purse your lips and blow a long, smooth breath into the palm of your hand. Keep this up for at least five more breaths.

Notice that if you're rushing this, breathing too fast, you start to feel light-headed. Wait until you feel a genuine need to breathe in before starting again. If, on the other hand, you've been breathing more slowly than usual, you might have noticed a calming effect.

The ancient yogis knew this calming effect and wrote about it at least 500 years ago. I've been very fortunate to train in a yoga tradition that has deep roots and in which the art of breathing has been preserved. However, today, what you've just been doing is one of the exercises recommended by the NHS in the UK and by the American Lung Association for people with breathing difficulty.

Yes, that's right! If you breathe out slowly, creating a little resistance at your pursed lips, your inner air passages stay inflated and your lungs extract more oxygen from each breath. Breathe slower, get more oxygen!

Was that so difficult? Often, if we have a problem with anything, our breath, our life even, we fear that any intervention will actually make things worse. In the short term, this is not an unreasonable fear. That's why, in this book, I have broken down the changes you need to make into small, safe steps.

EXERCISE 1.2: Sitting comfortably and watching your breath. First, find a comfortable upright sitting position that is right for you. If you're a yoga teacher trying this out, you may want to assume one of the two floor-sitting positions, but with enough support that your hips are above your knees. If you're going to sit on a support, choose a stool or a firm chair – sitting away from its back.

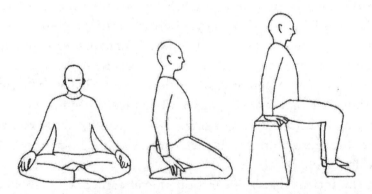

Figure 1: Three possible sitting positions for upright breathing, knees level with or below hips. If on a chair, ensure your feet are supported

Rest one hand in the other, relax your shoulders and close, or half-close your eyes. Simply watch your breath. You may feel a little nervous about this at first, but there is no need. After all, your breath is working for you 24 hours a day, though you hardly ever notice it. So, trust your breath now!

If you were able to breathe comfortably through your nose in the last exercise, that is the ideal. However, the next exercise is an interim outbreath-slowing exercise to be followed ONLY until you can easily and comfortably breathe out slowly through your nose.

EXERCISE 1.3: Focusing on a pursed-lip out-breath. Breathe in freely and immediately breathe out through pursed lips in a fine, gentle stream of air. Keep this up for about six breaths and then remain sitting quietly while you watch your breath return to its natural rhythm.

Breathing out rapidly through your mouth is NOT recommended; if this has become a habit with you, please be patient with this. Continue reading and following the exercises until you no longer feel the need to do this. Otherwise, breathing out slowly is your first priority. The second is to exhale through your nose, as soon as this is comfortable.

Perhaps you've read this far and said to yourself, 'Yes, I already know all this.' Or maybe the idea that changing the way you breathe could affect how you feel or even improve your health is new to you. Your breath wants to give you as near optimum health as it can. But for many of us, habits we've developed in the course of life can get in the way of relaxed breathing.

Whether you're already experienced at working with your breath, or a complete beginner, there will be something in this book for you. Please trust your breath to work in the best way it can and keep working with each exercise until it feels natural.

Two personal stories

Early in 2020, it dawned on the world that we were facing a new threat. On 23 March, the Government of the UK pretty much closed us down. No cars on the roads, no planes in the sky. Beautifully quiet, but no yoga classes allowed!

So, I went online and presented some courses consisting of seven weekly breathing classes. After all, we were facing what is basically a respiratory illness. As well as anxiety, stemming from the uncertainty which we were all facing, some people who attended had longstanding breathing issues. Here's what one of them said, after completing my course of seven weekly lessons:

Dear Michael, First of all, thank you so much for your excellent breathing classes. I have now incorporated the exercises into my daily yoga routine. I can't believe that having practised yoga most of my adult life I have paid so little attention to breathing. I was diagnosed as a mild asthmatic decades ago and my wheeze has now gone!
Vicky

It's likely that Vicky isn't unique and that there are millions of others who can be helped with just some simple exercises. I'm not saying that yoga breathing can provide an instant cure-all. However, the sheer range of ways of working with the breath that yoga provides makes it very likely that with persistence, imagination and, ideally, the help of a qualified teacher, significant improvements can be made.

Here's a longer story from someone else who attended my online classes. I hope that her story will help answer the question 'Why learn to breathe?'

Dear Michael, In October of 2020, we went to a cabin and our son and two young grandchildren were next door. We had booked a cycling slot at one of the centres. The cycling was quite challenging as we made several hill-starts behind our small grandson who had to stop and push his bike upwards.

At the top of a hill, I had to drop my bike as I had a pain in my chest and my diaphragm felt immovable – that is how it felt.

I feel that all of your discourse and physical practice with us meant that I didn't panic. I told myself to relax and concentrated on my breathing, which was difficult at first!! I used shallow breathing to start with and gradually my diaphragm seemed to move again.

My husband sent for an ambulance as I still had the pain in my chest and had gone grey, he said. I felt very tired and unable to use energy to speak while trying to work with my breathing.

I was tested in hospital but the tests did not flag up anything worrying and I was released after a few hours. Our own doctor repeated one or two tests when I saw her and, fortunately, there have not been any repercussions. Sudden over exertion was undoubtedly a factor but I do feel that the lack of panic and being able to help myself definitely helped.

The key point for me is that, while waiting rather a long time for an ambulance, I didn't get too stressed and was able to help myself, all thanks to your work and years of involvement with yoga.

My student still feels embarrassed about this incident which took place in front of her son and grandchildren and involved our overstretched medical services, but it could have been much worse. I believe now that she was suffering from diaphragm fatigue, which according to Patrick McKeown (2021, p163) can affect even top athletes. You will find more personal stories of my own and my students' as we go through this book, especially in Chapter 2.

Simple physiology

Our bodies need to take in oxygen and release carbon dioxide. This exchange is key to the process of respiration, which is fundamental to life. It has both an external aspect, which we experience as breathing, and an internal aspect, where oxygen is exchanged for carbon dioxide within all the tissues of our bodies.

As you know, it is your blood which carries oxygen to all these tissues. However, were you aware that you need carbon dioxide in your blood almost as much as you need oxygen? If you blow off too much carbon dioxide through rapid shallow breathing, then your body tissues find it difficult to extract oxygen from your blood.

This effect, discovered by Dr Christian Bohr in 1904, is the physiology behind panic attacks, since anxious shallow breathing depletes your blood of carbon dioxide. Your brain then cannot get as much oxygen as it needs. You will feel confused and breathless, but more shallow breathing will only make things worse. Unless someone like a doctor or paramedic intervenes, you may even collapse. Those of us who are habitual shallow breathers are more at risk of these distressing and embarrassing episodes.

There are three simple things that you can learn and which have been taken for granted by yogis for centuries.

1. Always breathe through your nose, except when speaking, singing, yawning, laughing or breathing out through pursed lips as described above.
2. Take some time to practise breathing out slowly, through your nose if you can. Set aside a couple of minutes two or three times a day, at least, to devote to breathing in freely and breathing out slowly.
3. Also, train yourself during these exercises to wait for a few seconds before breathing in each time.

In starting these exercises, you may be aiming to break the breathing habits of a lifetime. This means you will need to be patient and persistent, because any change will take weeks or months. Even if you start feeling better, you must keep up the exercises. As our teacher, Mr Desikachar, told us, the old, underlying patterns will be with you for quite a while, just waiting to take over again. If you persist, the results will be well worthwhile, even life-changing.

I mentioned earlier the patients with inexplicable symptoms whom other doctors were sending to cardiologist Dr Claude Lum. In many cases, Dr Lum found that, if patients persisted with breathing exercises, their symptoms sometimes improved dramatically. This shows that the effectiveness of breathing exercises was proven, in a medical setting, decades ago. However, even the simple 'Papworth' exercises (Holloway & West, 2007) which Dr Lum devised are still not applied very widely today. The same can be said of the exercises devised by Professor Dr Konstantin Buteyko, which focus on the third of my points, which is to develop the capacity to pause between breaths.

Replacing mouth breathing

By far the most problematic form of incorrect breathing is mouth breathing. To his excellent book on the Buteyko method, McKeown (2004) gave the simple title 'Close Your Mouth'. When I began training as a yoga teacher in 1983, breathing through the nose was simply stated as a requirement. This meant that, from then on, I was working on breaking any personal tendency to mouth breathing, at least during my own yoga practice.

However, mouth breathing as a habit did continue to creep back in, especially when I was feeling stressed. This was the last thing I needed to happen! Incorrect breathing patterns are, in their own way, trying to help when we feel stressed, but they do harm rather than good. When stressed, pausing every so often to take a few slower, deeper breaths not only helped to clear my mind, but also helped to gradually replace those bad habits.

Of course, if you are a really persistent mouth breather, it will be quite a step to switch all at once to breathing entirely through your nose. In fact, as McKeown points out, if you're not using your nose to breathe, it may become congested for that reason alone. In that case, where do we start? We need to break the problem down.

EXERCISE 1.4: Introducing a pause between breaths. Once you've been regularly repeating Exercise 1.3 you can begin to *pause* for a couple of seconds before letting the next breath in. For one thing, this slow breathing with a slight pause will be calming. Secondly, by breathing out slowly through the lips, the mouth and throat will become less dry.

Initially, the important thing is to slow your breath down. This will reduce the need to breathe through the mouth and also make it more likely that air will start to flow in your nose once it isn't blocked entirely. Four other things may help.

1. There'll be less suction on your nostrils from too-rapid airflow.
2. You may start yawning, helping you to relax.
3. Yawning may increase activity in your tear ducts, as will the abdominal breathing which you're about to learn (Sano et al, 2015).
4. Humming softly, just strongly enough to feel a gentle vibration in your head, alternating with gentle in-breaths – through your nose if you can.

Some yoga exercises will have a long-term clearing effect on the nasal passages. These include:

- Repeated forward bending, an exercise you will find in most yoga classes. If you have sinus discomfort, drop your head only until you get a feeling of fullness in your face. At first, this may mean you can only bend forward to touch a chair seat, your head just below your heart.

- Exercises that generate heat in the body will help to clear the nostrils. These could include the more dynamic, opening forms of yoga bodywork, postures and movements, where there is some physical demand but you can still either speak or breathe out through your nose.
- Making a firmer humming sound, so that you can really feel the vibration in your head. This will also stimulate the release of nitric oxide gas (NO), a natural purifier produced in healthy sinuses.
- Firm massage of the muscles where your head joins your neck; tightness here can exacerbate sinus congestion.

When learning to breathe through your nose again, it is important never to sniff your breath in. The very act of sniffing restricts the passage of air. Rapid air movement tends to cause constriction, this is known in physics as the Venturi effect. If you try to inhale rapidly through your nose, without sniffing, you will still feel a light pulling in at the pinch pit of your nostrils.

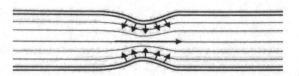

Figure 2. The Venturi effect happens at a pinch point in a tube through where the air has to speed up to get through. This speeding up causes a drop in pressure at the pinch point, pulling the walls of the tube in further

Training yourself to breathe more slowly and deeply will also help you to take a big step away from mouth breathing. Sniffing your breath out, on the other hand, doesn't cause as much restriction and just a few gentle sniffs can have a clearing effect. Pause afterward, until a need to breathe in is felt distinctly.

Relearning nose breathing can be a challenge. In which case, it may help you to consider that while horses are obligate nose breathers and cannot mouth-breathe, they can run for miles at 30mph (50kph) and sprint at 40mph (65kph). I remember watching the Boxing Day races on TV with my late father-in-law many years ago. Stan had grown up between the wars in the Berkshire Downs – horse-training country. In the frosty late December air, it was plain to see that each horse was breathing in time with its own stride, that is OUT when its front and back legs were being drawn together and consequently IN when they were stretched forward and back. In the next chapter, you'll be invited to get on all-fours and explore yourself the relationship between breathing and spinal movement – but at rest, not at 30mph!

Once you start to get some regular airflow in your nose, you will start to notice more of the smells around you, feel the fresh air and enjoy your food more. Additionally, the world of regular yoga breathing exercises will then be open to you.

Ease and patience

Perhaps the most important single piece of advice is to work with your breath with ease and patience. Your breath is with you every moment of your life and in a sense is your closest and most important friend. This is why work with the breath should never be a struggle; it is vital never to try to force the breath to work in a certain way. Yogi Svātmārāma (fifteenth century) (ā is pronounced long, as in 'calm') wrote that working with the breath was like taming an elephant, lion or tiger. That means we must work gently and with caution, with respect and with the idea that our breath is our friend, one to be encouraged to work in ways that will help us.

The flow of breath which we are seeking to experience is quiet and slow. We want no noise to distract us from the subtle coolness of the breath as it comes in, or from its gentle warmth as it flows out. Mr Desikachar (1999, p56) said that, 'We must acutely sense and feel the movement of the breath within.' This is where yoga breathing, as distinct from exercises with the breath, really begins. It is vital to yoga and similar disciplines.

EXERCISE 1.5: Watching your breath in a lying position. An important way of learning patience, which all my students seem to enjoy, is to simply lie down and watch your breath. The classic yoga position of rest is to lie fully stretched out, arms and legs straight but not rigid. Have your legs slightly apart and let your toes on each side rest outwards. Rest your arms a little way from your sides, with your palms turned away from the floor. You may need a little head support.

If your lower back starts to feel tight in this position, try having a soft bolster under your knees. If that's not enough, draw your feet in closer to the body, knees raised. Finally, it's possible to rest your lower legs and feet on the seat of a chair, with a cushion, if need be.

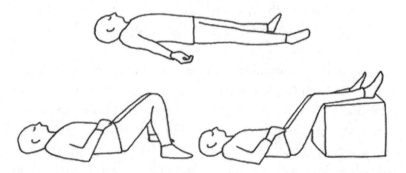

Figure 3: Three possible lying positions for resting breathing

Letting-go below

We shall be looking at active abdominal breathing in the next chapter. For now, and maybe to prepare for it, we can try just passive abdominal breathing.

EXERCISE 1.6: Passive abdominal breathing with resting hands. For this exercise, the crook-lying position, (middle position in Figure 3) with a little support under the head, and possibly a blanket over the knees to help the legs to relax, is the one you may find most helpful. Or you could rest your lower legs on a chair or stool; it's very important to be relaxed for this exercise. Place your hands over the tummy and invite your breath to flow in as deeply as it can, so you feel some lifting under your hands. This may be only slight at first, but as you relax and release, the effect will grow stronger. The exhale can be passive; all you need to feel is your tummy slowly sinking back in.

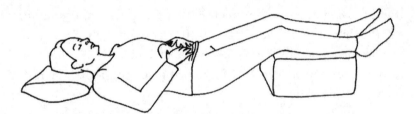

Figure 4: Feeling the rise and passive fall of the abdominal wall in relaxed, lying breathing

This passive abdominal breathing is certainly therapeutic. In 2010, I met Juraj Gajdos, www.jogagajdos.sk, a former member of the Slovenian soccer team, when we were both teaching at the European Yoga Congress in Switzerland. He assured us that this deep abdominal breathing, learnt from the team's yoga teacher, had helped him recover from a serious back injury suffered on the soccer pitch.

EXERCISE 1.7: Passive abdominal breathing with arms spread. If abdominal breathing doesn't come easily, lying work will be a much easier way for you to begin. There's one more step that could help you to trigger this mode of breathing. In the crook-lying position (middle position in Figure 3), rest your arms by your sides. Each time you breathe in, slide your hands and arms along the floor a little further out to the sides, thus expanding your ribs. Gradually, you will start to feel your breath going in deeper. As you relax and start to feel more at peace, watching your breath, you may start to experience that feeling I call 'breathfulness'.

Your respiratory diaphragm

If you're already familiar with the anatomy of breathing, you won't need to read this section. Nor will you need to think about the anatomy in this section while you're doing the exercises, since we can't feel our respiratory diaphragms, only the breathing movements they create. Otherwise, this section will help you to understand how your diaphragm works. As one of my students recently said:

> Dear Michael, I felt after your seminar yesterday that teaching people about their respiratory anatomy and physiology will be really useful to help understand why we are doing what we do with yoga. It really helps to put the importance of the breath into context and I think it can only help people take responsibility for their health when they understand their body more.
> Jane.

I've been using terms like abdominal breathing to talk about somewhere in the body we can feel movement from the action of our breath. As I'm sure you're already aware, air does not enter your abdominal area when you inhale. Your body is divided between your upper (chest) cavity and your lower (abdominal) cavity by a sheet of muscle and connective tissue called the respiratory diaphragm. When relaxed, after you've breathed out, it's a little like a mushroom with its roots on the inside of your lower back:

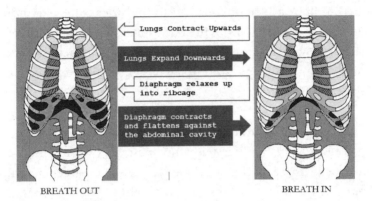

BREATH OUT   BREATH IN

Figure 5: Illustration of the lungs (pale grey) and diaphragm (dark grey on top, mid-grey underneath) and where they sit in relation to the body on both exhale (left) and inhale (right). Where the diaphragm lies under the lower ribs, its outline is shown dotted. The diaphragm is also shaded paler where it's behind the ribs. The hatched areas each side of the breastbone will be explained in Chapter 4

As you inhale, your diaphragm will contract and flatten, pushing against your abdominal organs to make room for more air to enter your lungs. You won't feel your diaphragm working; however, you can feel its effect in the way your tummy pushes outwards as your breath fills in a relaxed way. This manner of using your diaphragm, which also includes a gentle outward expansion of your ribs, is the least effortful and most relaxed way to breathe. Very young children breathe this way naturally.

The following diagrams show a side view of how the diaphragm descends and flattens as it contracts. Tone in the abdominal wall keeps the lower organs supported. Also, nerve impulses will tell the diaphragm it has a restorative force against which it can push on inhaling. Without this gentle tone providing compression from below, there would be nothing to lift your diaphragm back into its expanded, breath-out position (left in Figure 5) so it will not descend in the first place.

Something that Mr Desikachar observed many years ago, and which I often see, is the way that people breathe better when lying down. This is because their diaphragms can then work fully, even in the absence of abdominal muscle coordination, because gravity is there to push down and return their diaphragms back into their chests. Please have a look at Figure 6.

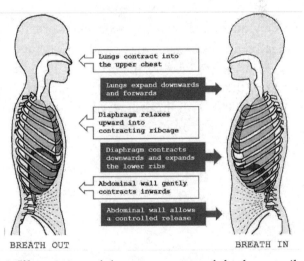

Figure 6: Illustration of the movements of the lungs, ribs and diaphragm between the breath-out and breath-in positions

Perhaps lie down now and re-connect with the lifting and lowering of your tummy as you breathe in and out, as in the two previous exercises, feeing how gravity helps your breath to flow out. If you find that you lose this capacity to make full use of your diaphragm when you sit up or stand, the exercises that follow will help you to restore it. At first, you will need to ask consciously for your abdominal wall muscles to respond, using the exercises in the following chapter.

EXERCISES SUMMARY CHAPTER 1:
1.1 Blowing into the palm of your hand
1.2 Sitting comfortably and watching your breath
1.3 Focusing on a pursed-lip out-breath
1.4 Introducing a pause between breaths
1.5 Watching your breath in a lying position
1.6 Passive abdominal breathing with resting hands
1.7 Passive abdominal breathing with arms spread

Step-by-step – 1

Before moving on, be sure you now feel able to breathe out more slowly, ideally through your nose, and pause for a moment between breaths. Also, be sure that you can feel, in a relaxed lying position, the rise and fall of your tummy with your in- and out-breaths. This will mean that you're ready for my next chapter.

Chapter 2

Exhale Slowly

When emerging from a stressful experience, we will often exhale rapidly – phew! Fine as this is for an occasional release, it creates no other relaxation in the system. This is the current online advice from Harvard Medical School:

> Find a quiet, comfortable place to sit or lie down. First, take a normal breath. Then try a deep breath: Breathe in slowly through your nose, allowing your chest and lower belly to rise as you fill your lungs. Let your abdomen expand fully. Now breathe out slowly through your mouth (or your nose, if that feels more natural).
> Harvard Medical School, July 2020

However, I'd have preferred it if they'd simply said 'breathe out slowly through your nose', because that IS what's natural, regardless of any life-habits, or even some exercise methods that promote mouth exhalation. Slow exhalation through your nose helps your lungs, contracting slowly, to work more effectively.

Simple movement

A simple and direct way to slow the breath down is to synchronise breath and movement. Somehow, getting the body involved feels more natural, less stressed, than focusing on the breath alone. Also, movements can mirror the length and even, as we shall see, the structure of the breath.

EXERCISE 2.1: Lifting the hands off the heart as you inhale. Standing or sitting in a comfortable, upright position, rest your hands over your heart, as on the left in Figure 7 below.

As you feel your breath coming in, lift your hands away, just a short distance for now. Return your hands to your heart as you breathe out. Can you feel your breath wanting to tie in with these gentle opening and closing movements of the hands and arms? See if it's possible to ask the breath to be slow enough that it will last the whole movement, especially the return of the hands to the heart as you breathe out through your nose or pursed lips.

For now, it doesn't matter whether you breathe through your nose or not. However, nose breathing will get easier if you can make the breath slower and deeper. See if you can let your breath into your belly. Deeper breathing gets the lungs working more efficiently and also helps the heart to work more easily. But if not, don't be concerned, we can come back to that when you're ready. Here's what one of my students has said about the value of coordinated breathing and movement:

> I have been going to Michael's yoga classes for many years. I find them very therapeutic for both body and mind. Michael's use of breath with movement helps to de-stress the mind and loosen the body in a way nothing else does in these fast-paced times. Michael is a fantastic teacher and always observes individuals to ensure movements are carried out correctly. He is highly thought of by his many students as well as having an outstanding reputation in the yoga world. If you are looking for peace of mind and soul look no further.
> Alison

EXERCISE 2.2: Movement and breath: easy standing forward bend. Let's make that breath-body coordination into the short sequence in Figure 7. Lift your hands off your heart, breathing in, but lift them higher. As you breathe out, bend forward a little to place your hands on your thighs, neck relaxed. Pause for a moment, then as you start to breathe in, lift your hands. Let your lifting hands and incoming breath lead you into the upright, arms raised position. Exhale slowly, returning your hands to your heart. When we become absorbed in this mindful flow of breath and movement, we feel peaceful and this feeling becomes something we want to experience again.

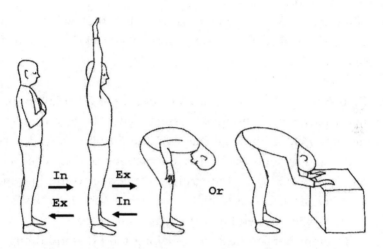

Figure 7. Easy standing forward bend sequence
(can also be taken sitting)

This peaceful, mindful, breathfulness is in fact an experience of yoga and it's so simple, with no headstand or sitting cross-legged required. Yet, if you're attentively coordinating the movement of the breath with that of the body, it is more truly yoga than if you were to twist your body into some complicated posture, only to neglect your breath. However, simple isn't always the same as easy. As soon as your attention wanders, as soon as your breath and your body movements cease to be coordinated, it stops being yoga and that feeling of inner peace drifts away.

The challenge is to remain attentive, and in yoga we have ways and means to hold our attention. There are many, many movements and postures and many, many ways of working with the breath, so we can always find something new to engage our attention. *However, yoga is about experience, not achievement, not a list of things to accomplish.* It is certainly not about any striving or strain. But sometimes, without being conscious of trying, we will find ourselves doing something we could not do before. That, also, is yoga.

Sometimes my students pass on what they've learnt to help friends and family. Here is some feedback I received in December 2021:

Dear Michael, my mum suffers from Atrial Fibrillation and in the past would end up in hospital, where they couldn't do much to help. I think she has it all the time but only notices it at night, when there are less distractions, and so when she would feel her heart thumping at 2am, she would become anxious and this would make it worse, so much so that she would sometimes end up calling an ambulance.

I taught her long exhale – making the exhalation longer than the inhalation. She also uses Ujjāyī and Kara Nyāsa when she feels anxious. She finds that after 10–15 minutes of using this breath, her AF calms down to bearable levels and she can get to sleep. This has empowered her to manage the AF herself and given her confidence that she is in control of her breathing, and through this, the AF itself. Merry Christmas!
Patricia.

Kara Nyāsa is like a simple ritual to calm yourself by breathing in time with a sequence of finger movements. Ujjāyī is a technique of slowing the breath by creating a soft restriction in the throat. I shall provide you with instruction in both Ujjāyī and Kara Nyāsa in later chapters.

Simple sounds

When our distant ancestors became able to slow their out-breaths, this opened up the possibility of making an extended series of sounds to convey meaning. At the same time, not having to spend hours chewing uncooked foods meant that their mouths could became more adapted to speech (Wrangham, 2009). The result is that we modern humans are capable of making a far wider range of sounds than any of our far-distant ancestors.

Speech, making sounds and lengthening the out-breath remain closely linked. As soon as we even think about making sounds, the breath becomes ready to slow down. Earlier, we explored breathing out slowly through pursed lips. We can add a soft 'OOO' sound to this (written as Ū, a capital U with a bar above). Try this now:

EXERCISE 2.3: Introducing the Ū sound in a gentle, wide-legged twist. In a quiet place by yourself, stand with your feet 30-40 cm apart, shoulders relaxed. Close your eyes and breathe in freely. Purse the lips and make a soft, long Ū sound. Pause for a moment, then breathe in freely again. Keep this up for about 12 breaths, then make sure to allow some free breaths.

Now you can get moving with this. Place your hands on your tummy. As you breathe in, ease one hand slowly round to its own side and follow it with your gaze, bringing a gentle twist into your whole body. As you breathe out with the Ū sound, slowly return to facing the front, bringing your hand back to rest on the other hand. Slip your underneath hand out as you breathe in to repeat to the other side. Allow yourself to be free and soft in your body so you feel a gentle twist from head to feet. Continue repeating to alternate sides for up to 10 more breaths, never hurrying and easing slowly into the last bit of the turn.

Please avoid any 'ballistic' work, which uses the elasticity of the body to stop movements. This has in my own experience caused strain in my upper back.

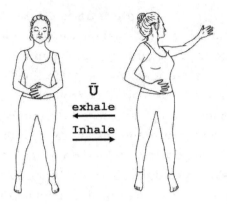

Figure 8. Upright standing twist/stretch, returning with pursed lips

You may have noticed the long Ū sound you were making was varying in strength. One of the benefits of making a sound is we get to know how smooth and consistent the breath is, or could be. Which is more pleasant to hear, a singer whose voice is wavering, or one whose voice is smooth and clear? We enjoy the latter more because a clear and steady sound also tells us that the singer is more confident and relaxed. From a respiratory perspective, a smooth steady exhale is more effective, but also making a smooth out-breath is more calming. This means we can use a soft sound with the out-breath to gauge our progress towards having that smooth, calm, confident breath. I hinted in the section on clearing the nose (see Exercise 1.4 and what follows) that making a firm humming sound could help. Let's try that now. I will be writing the sound like this: Ṃ, a capital M with a dot below.

EXERCISE 2.4: Clearing the head with a humming sound Ū-Ṃ. In a quiet place, sit in a comfortable upright sitting position, with relaxed shoulders, as in Exercise 1.4. Try 12 Ṃ out-breaths with free inhalations. Or you can play around by combining the two to make a long Ū-Ṃ. If this practice has induced some mental quiet, relax and stay with that for a minute or two.

In my work as a yoga therapist, I often play around until my student and I find a sound that produces the feeling, effect or experience that we are looking for. Often, initial embarrassment about making sounds causes a fair bit of amusement, but there's no harm in that.

Very occasionally, a student of mine has become tearful. If in the past you have reined in your expression of some grief or pain, your body and also your breath will hold this pain in the form of unconscious tension and restriction. Exercises like this can sometimes bring about an unexpected release, especially if a supportive person is present. It is then the job of such people to encourage you to release. With their help you can both see and experience an opportunity for release by breathing and relaxing your way through it. Neither you nor your teacher, therapist or helper should be in any hurry to work out the cause of your tears; this will reveal itself in time.

Abdominal exhalation

Thinking about simple sounds leads us to an important exercise that I have, for many years, been teaching to help people to breathe out more positively, fully and effectively, a method that brings, along with it, other benefits. You will be encouraging an *active* abdominal out-breath, which is a step on from the passive abdominal breathing that you practised in Chapter 1. The muscles that pull your tummy in are called the transverse abdominals and are hard to re-activate other than by working with your breath.

EXERCISE 2.5: Engaging your transverse abdominals with sounds Ū or M. You will need to be either down on your hands and knees or, if that's not easy or comfortable, standing with your hands about level with your knees and resting on the seat of a chair in front of you, as in the lower part of Figure 9. In either case, have your hips directly over your knees and your wrists a little forward of the points directly under your shoulders.

If you are on your knees, it's good to have a little padding to make sure they're comfortable. In all cases, keep your shoulders relaxed away from your ears. It may help initially to have someone watch you, since many of my students have found this exercise is not as simple as it looks.

You are going to be making a movement on your out-breath. Your hips will go back, your head will gently drop and you will feel a release in your *lower* back as you look between your knees. If you are kneeling, your knees will be bending a little more. Note that your upper back must stay flat, as in Figure 9, and *not* round into a 'Cow' pose. On your in-breath, you will come back to the starting position, shoulders eased back, looking at your fingertips.

Why do people want to round their upper backs? It's a question Mr Desikachar used to ask. While it can release tension there, the real answer to a tight upper back, which I shall reveal in Chapter 4, lies in the front of the body.

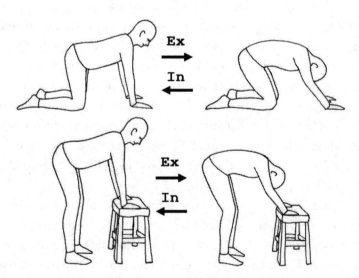

Figure 9: Easy kneeling or standing movement back and forth between breath in with front of body open (left) and breath out with front of body closed (right)

Once you've got the hang of the movement and can coordinate it with your breath, start making the long Ū sound with your out-breath and backwards movement. What we are looking for, the feeling, effect or experience, is the 'tummy', the abdominal wall, lifting in towards the spine. It's OK to just keep asking for this to happen. The movement, the sound, the pursing of the lips, the closing of the throat, these are all triggers for the contraction of the transverse abdominal muscles. If the Ū sound isn't helping, try the Ṃ instead. Feel free to play around!

This is not a recommendation for everyone, but when I had a hernia repair operation in 1990 (before keyhole surgery!) my then teacher, Paul Harvey, gave me this exercise to do every day, starting the day after the operation. Having to make the sound with the movement meant that I would be neither under- nor over-exerting in my abdominals. Please note that Paul's advice was for me individually at the time and is NOT a general prescription post-surgery!

To summarise, this exercise will:

- Strengthen and lengthen your out-breath
- Tone your abdominal muscles to the correct degree, with no straining
- Take you further towards habitual good use of your diaphragm
- Give some release to your lower back
- Possibly, release some emotional tension and feelings of being stressed

To demonstrate the healing potential for the breath of the use of sound, in 2020, the English National Opera ENO-Breathe initiative, in collaboration with Imperial College, UK, showed encouraging results from a trial with patients suffering with long-COVID-19 (Imperial College Healthcare, 2021).

The sound that you make doesn't have to be 'pretty'. I tell my students it's OK to make a sound like a foghorn, or the wind over the top of a drainpipe. Feel free to put some feeling into it and not worry about how it sounds! On the other hand, a very soft sound, or even a silent, mental Ū or M, can sometimes be the most effective. See what feels most releasing for you.

Here's a personal story about the power of abdominal breathing sent by a private student who found me online during the recent pandemic. While at first, I'd taught Jillian the above exercise using simple sounds, by this stage she no longer needed to make the sound to remind her out-breath to work from low down:

Dear Michael, I just wanted to say thank you for taking the time to teach me over the last year. The last few months have been quite a bit more stressful than normal and I can't tell you how many times your voice has popped into my head when I've tried to slow my anxious breathing! Thank you! At our last lesson, you had me inhale and exhale solely from my stomach and that actually helped me relax today; I'm currently sick and my breathing has been difficult for a few days. I've continued a light yoga practice, but I get out of breath easily and have to nearly chant to myself 'let my breath be my friend' :)
Thank you,
Jillian

I found it very heartening that Jillian could continue with her breathwork and even a light yoga practice while feeling unwell. We need never give up!

My own personal story about healing with sound dates from the 1990s, when I used to attend an annual Tantric chanting retreat led by Muz Murray www.muzmurray.com. I was at the time under investigation for a suspected gall bladder problem.

During one of the extended chanting sessions, the pain in this region intensified, but I carried on chanting. Suddenly, the pain seemed to dissolve and has never come back, even to this day.

Your lower back

Not only have you been powering your out-breath from below in the previous exercise, you were also creating tone in the 'core support' muscles that help maintain your posture. The transverse abdominal muscles which are activated in this way run round your sides and actually interleave with your lower back muscles. Therefore, these two sets of muscles are clearly meant to work together in supporting your lower back. But how does this work?

Remember, to breathe out we need to have positive pressure in the body which is trying to contract and close, so the air flows out. Some of this positive pressure comes from the fact that the body, including even the lungs themselves, is elastic, so what expands will contract on its own without effort. But the body can do more than simply be passive.

The core muscles can maintain an active, responsive tone. When the breath needs to come in, they can let go a little and then contract again when it's time to breathe out. If we have good resting tone in the core muscles, this will happen unconsciously, every time we breathe. Given this core tone, your breath will feel more confident about going in deeper, knowing that the abdominal wall will assist it on its way out. However, with time and the ups and downs of life, this linkage can get lost, even when we are young, hence the need for exercises like 2.5.

To support our lower back at certain times, such as lifting a load, what is needed is a slow, firm, throaty out-breath from below, gently engaging the core support muscles, which will create a positive pressure in the abdominal cavity. Figure 10 shows a cross-section through the abdomen and lower back, at the level of one of the spinal discs.

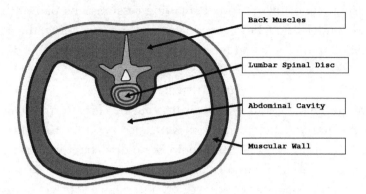

Figure 10: Simplified cross-section through the spine and abdomen, showing the small relative size of the spinal disc

For those of you who like maths, a typical lumbar disc is about 4 cm wide and about 3 cm front to back, so will have a load-bearing area of about 10 cm² or 0.001 m² (1.5 in²). The entire abdomen cavity is typically about 6 times wider and deeper, so its load-bearing area will be about 350 cm² or 0.035 m² (55 in²).

The pressure on each lumbar disc from supporting, for example, a 50kg load (25 kg weight plus 25 kg for the weight of the upper body, 55 lb+55lb) will therefore be about 50,000 kg/m² or about 70 psi, about twice the pressure in your car tyres!

Suppose then we pressurise the abdominal volume to just 1.0psi or 700 kg/m². This is only 7% of atmospheric pressure, yet it will supply an upward force of about 700 x 0.035 = 25 kg (55lb). We can see from this very rough example that it doesn't require much pressure from your diaphragm and your abdominal wall muscles to take about half the load off your lumbar discs.

This is how abdominal tone, as well as supporting your out-breath, helps to support your lower back. As one of my students reported recently:

Hi Michael, I found your teaching on how the breath provides an equal and opposite pressure for the core to press against useful. The model of 'seeing' my core muscles wrapping around the breath (as if taking air into the abdominal area) and therefore providing my core with something to work against (intra-abdominal pressure) during strength training, thus providing optimal support for the spine, and it makes you stronger structurally. So – in short – l am lifting heavier weights and have avoided injury – thank you.
Melissa.

However, it's not only the instances which we think of as load-bearing that count. For those with chronic spinal conditions, every movement can be a significant load-bearing event. One of my students who had been suffering chronic back pain and was reluctant to start yoga again wrote to me in November 2021 as follows:

Dear Michael,
I am very appreciative of you allowing me to share your weekly classes and helping to give me the confidence to be reunited with my yoga this year. It has meant a great deal to me. Now I just look to the future with a renewed energy and from this morning a new practice. Not only has yoga come back to me but yesterday I had my back consultation and was able to say my back is 50 per cent improved and, touch wood, without the awful pain I was experiencing.
Best wishes,
Steph

Furthermore, for years when teaching balance work, I've been suggesting that to maintain a gentle abdominal tone in these postures will help. Research (Hodges et al, 2005) has shown that a positive intra-abdominal pressure does indeed help. However, thinking of more everyday activities, here is an exercise which, if practised regularly, will help instil the habit of engaging the abdominal wall when bending forward. It's one of those simple everyday situations where the lower back has to work, if only to lift the upper body.

EXERCISE 2.6: Active abdominal out-breath in a standing forward bend. If, as shown in Figure 11, you're able to repeat Exercise 2.2 while making the sound Ū or M̩ in such a way as to trigger your abdominal tone, this will support your lower back in the forward bend and encourage it to release just a little more. Take it easy! Let your out-breath and your lower back talk to each other.

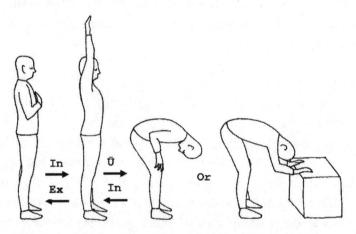

Figure 11. Easy standing forward bend sequence

The aim here is that, with daily practice, your core muscles will gently engage each time you bend forwards, protecting your back, without your having to think about it. You may have noticed, or be aware, that your pelvic floor muscles are contributing to the core tone you're feeling on exhalation. There is a lot of debate these days regarding ways to maintain the health of the pelvic floor.

Your pelvic floor

What I have learnt from my teachers and in the course of my own teaching and daily practice is that I am sharing with you the best way known to maintain your pelvic floor. Working in concert with your breath and voice, your pelvic floor will contract on every out-breath to about 30% of maximum. This is what Mr Desikachar advised and what my students, some of whom have experienced two or more vaginal births, have found helpful. For them, pelvic floor exercise is necessary; however, overly strong contractions can leave them with lingering and unnecessary discomfort. Furthermore, my female colleagues who regularly teach yoga for pregnancy have reported that pregnant women who have previously over-developed their pelvic floors can suffer more difficulty, pain and potential damage from a vaginal delivery.

The situation of those who, for whatever reason, have chronically tight pelvic floors must also be considered. Here, it is working with the in-breath that can be helpful. Starting a lying position, a downflow breath can be felt, with practice, in the pelvic bowl and even in the surrounding gluteal muscles.

EXERCISES SUMMARY CHAPTER 2:
2.1 Lifting the hands off the heart as you inhale
2.2 Movement and breath: easy standing forward bend
2.3 Introducing the Ū sound in a gentle, wide-legged twist
2.4 Clearing the head with a humming sound Ū-Ṃ
2.5 Engaging your transverse abdominals with sounds Ū or Ṃ
   in a prone position: active abdominal out-breath.
2.6 Active abdominal out-breath in a standing forward bend

Step-by-step – 2

You should now be able to combine breathing with simple movements. Being allowed to move made the exercises easier and more enjoyable for you. Also, you got used to making simple sounds and found this helpful and even releasing. The final exercise 2.6 was to test if your core muscles could, with a little encouragement, direct your breath up and out. This will mean that you're ready for the next chapter.

Chapter 3

Learn to Pause

In the exercises so far, you've been invited to pause after breathing out and then wait until you feel the need to breathe in again. As well as helping to increase your awareness of how your breath is working, this was also to ensure that you were not over-breathing. However, pausing between breaths is in itself an important part of learning breath control. In particular, a progressive approach to breath-pausing is part of breaking the cycle of anxiety and excessive or irregular breathing.

Pausing after each breath is a way of developing faith and confidence that the next breath will come in and will be sufficient for your needs. Naturally, you may be concerned you are not taking in enough oxygen, but there is no need to worry, unless you have a serious heart or lung condition. In which case, you should keep breath-pauses short.

At first, you may only be able to pause, to keep your breath out, for a moment. Keeping your core muscles gently toned inwards as you pause will not only help keep your breath out, but add to your feeling of confidence and gentle control.

Remember, you are turning your breath from a source of anxiety into a reservoir of confidence. Your breath is becoming your friend!

Waiting for the need

Maybe you started with a pattern of unconscious, over-rapid breathing, maybe with your nose being neglected. Now you have come to the point of realising that you can be patient with your breath, you can slow it down and start to pause between breaths.

EXERCISE 3.1: Trial pause between breaths. Assume whatever is your comfortable, upright sitting position, eyes closed. Breathe out, lifting your tummy in a little and pause with your breath out for 10 seconds (or 5 seconds, if you have a heart or lung condition).

If lifting the tummy in (what I call the abdominal in-lift) is still something you can only do now and then, precede your pause with a long Ū exhale to stimulate your inner abs. Sit quietly through the pause, then let a few free breaths happen. It's important after any exercise with your breath to let it just go back to its own gentle rhythm for a while. Remember, you are being friendly with your breath!

With practice, your diaphragm and your core muscles will relearn to work in concert as you breathe. We saw earlier that, as your breath comes in, your core muscles need to soften to allow room for your diaphragm to descend. When it's time to exhale, the same core muscles will increase their tone to restore your abdominal wall to its resting position, once your diaphragm has relaxed upward into your chest cavity.

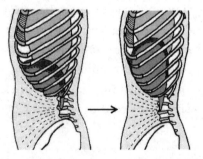

Figure 12. The abdominal in-lift is mostly created by your transverse abdominal muscles (fibres indicated by dashed lines) which shorten to pull your tummy in round your sides towards your back. Your internal oblique and anterior pelvic floor muscles assist with this action. The range of movement shown is somewhat exaggerated, relative to relaxed, quiet breathing.

As we saw earlier, learning this 'downflow' mode of inhaling can be easier when lying supine, because gravity does the job of the core muscles. To continue this downflow breathing when you sit or stand upright, begin by repeating Exercise 3.1 every day. It will cultivate both gentle core tone and its reciprocal working relationship with your diaphragm.

Perhaps you can see now why downflow breathing was introduced when you were resting on your back, where gravity provided the restorative force to balance the contraction of your diaphragm as you inhaled. However, there wouldn't have been much point in leaving you there. What you need is for your downflow breathing to continue after you've sat up. In too many people, it stops.

You now have the means to continue your downflow breathing in a sitting or standing position, even if you need to practise it consciously at first. Work gently, though, the contraction of these core support muscles must not be overdone. Learning to engage them while making a soft, smooth, deep sound will ensure the correct level of engagement, about 30% of maximum. More isn't always better!

To return to the idea of waiting for the need to inhale, we can now make this pause part of a rhythm or pattern with the breath:

EXERCISE 3.2: Maintaining a repeated pause between breaths, extending from 2 to 4 seconds. Breathe inwards and downwards freely, through your nose if possible. Exhale slowly, making or thinking a soft Ū sound if help is needed to lift your tummy in. Pause for just 2 seconds. Continue with this for at least 6 breaths.

If this feels too easy, then without a break extend your pause to 4 seconds and see how that feels after a second round of 6 breaths.

Work for another 6 breaths, making your pause longer, but not as long as it takes you to breathe out. Your in-breath should stay free and also take less time than does breathing out.

After this third round of 6 breaths, let your breath be completely free, while still giving it your full attention, for at least 6 more breaths.

You've just been doing some structured breathwork; however, focusing on the free breath can be very relaxing. If you're able to take a comfortable lying position as in Exercise 1.5, close your eyes and just watch your breath going in and out. Asking your breath to pause for a moment before coming in each time can be for you a moment of complete stillness.

Turning your breath around

Teaching classes for many years, I've noticed now and then that some people, when asked to focus on their breathing, will close their throats between inhale and exhale, or even between exhale and inhale. It makes their breath sound like it's turning a sharp corner when shifting from in to out. It's quite unnecessary and introduces tension into the throat. One thing we definitely don't want in our work with our breath is any tightness or tension.

It's helpful, then, to visualise the flow of your breath gradually tapering off towards the end of the in-breath and the flow gradually resuming in the opposite direction. In the visualisation, it's more like your breath is making a smooth, round loop at each end, like the smooth curve in Figure 13, rather than the sharp or sudden dashed angles.

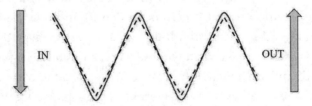

IN   OUT

Figure 13. Breathing in and out with time, with either sharp or smooth turn-rounds

EXERCISE 3.3: You can combine this pausing between breaths with movement, lifting your arms with your in-breath and lowering with your out-breath, as in Figure 14. When you do this, your arms copy or provide a template for what you want to experience with the breath, so the turn-around of their movement must also be smooth. Try this now, feeling the movement of both your breath and your arms tapering off slowly and then just as slowly starting off in the opposite direction.

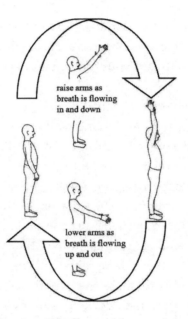

raise arms as
breath is flowing
in and down

lower arms as
breath is flowing
up and out

Figure 14. Coordinating inhaling with opening, arm-lifting and exhaling with closing, arm-lowering. Can also be done seated

When you first started coordinating breath and movement, it's likely that your breath, either out or back in, didn't quite last the whole movement it was meant to follow. However, if you're now able to complete this exercise, it shows that your breath and coordination have significantly improved.

Stay with this exercise of encouraging your breath to last the whole movement. Do not be concerned if your turn-around of your breath isn't perfect. Relax and this will come with practice, but please be sure you're comfortable with it before going to the next stage.

Breath > Movement

Progressing beyond the exercises so far, you're now ready for something that will serve you well in whatever practice you have, so long as it involves coordination of breath and movement.

So far, your coordination has probably been such that your breath and your movement have been in what I call 'lockstep'. That is, your breath and your movement both begin and end at the same moment.

Once you have mastered this, it becomes too easy to keep up this coordination without having to think about it. Your mind can wander and you will find that you've been continuing to breathe and move on a sort of 'autopilot'.

This may be okay from an exercise point of view, but it is NOT yoga. For an exercise to be yoga, or an alternative discipline such as Tai Chi, for example, your attention must be continuous and uninterrupted by any other train of thought.

While I am talking here about being mindful, what I really want to do is to share the experience of having breath, movement and attention working side-by-side with a deep sense of involvement. I'm talking about a mindfulness that is supported by a sense of breathfulness.

If, instead of breath and movement being in lockstep, what happens when we break this 'lockstep'? What if we resolve to start the breath first, then a moment later the movement that goes with it? And if we then complete both the breath and the movement, now running in parallel, and finish the movement, but still have a little breath left to go?

This mental separation of breath and movement can be done on both inhale and exhale, but it's easier to learn it first on the out-breath. Let's try this, just with the arms raising and lowering as you've done before.

EXERCISE 3.4: Exhale longer than Movement (or EX>MM): Breathe in and while doing so lift your arms, shoulders relaxed. Start to breathe out, just for a moment, keeping your arms raised. Feel your tummy lift in slightly. Once your outflow of breath is established, lower your arms, aiming to have a little breath left to flow out once your arms have come to rest. Raise your arms again, inhaling, as in the previous exercise. Repeat the cycle at least five more times.

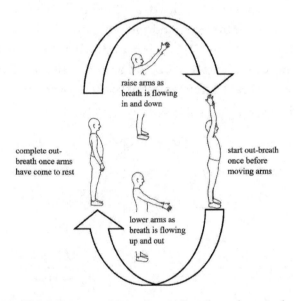

Figure 15. EX>MM; arm-lowering is bracketed entirely within the out-breath. Can also be done seated

Mr Desikachar used to write this as: Breath>Movement, or just BR>MM

At times when you let your attention wander, you will have realised, when you brought it back, that your out-breath and the return of the arms to the sides had gone back into 'lockstep'. But while you were able to keep up the parallel flow of movement, breath and attention, you will have experienced the feeling of mindful involvement that I call breathfulness, where the whole experience seems to ride on the breath.

When we aim for BR>MM, it never fails to catch us out, IF we let our attention wander. When you've truly established this on your out-breath and feel ready to move on, you can also practise BR>MM on your inhale movements.

EXERCISE 3.5: Both Exhale & Inhale > Movement. While you are lifting your arms, aim to have a little space left for more air once your arms are fully raised. With your arms and shoulders relaxed, turn your breath round smoothly from in to out and then start to lower the arms again, breath flowing out smoothly the whole time. Complete with EX>MM as in Exercise 3.4, but start to feel a little in-breath before you start to lift the arms again. Repeat the cycle at least 5 more times, as shown in Figure 16.

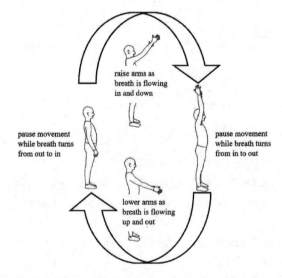

Figure 16. Exhale, breath escapes upwards, arms lower. Breath turns around, arms pause. Inhale, breath flows down, arms up. Breath turns around, arms pause

Simple, but to remember it, you need to keep very focused! But once you have it, this way of breath and movement coordination can be applied whatever your practice is like, so long as it requires coordination of breath and movement.

Moments of inner stillness

You may be aware that the key definition of yoga, at the start of Srī Patañjali's 'Yoga Sūtra', is that yoga is the stilling of the mind. Most of the time, if we have nothing useful to occupy the mind, it will fill itself with all sorts of daydreams, worries and imaginings. Our practice of yoga (including that of meditation), or of Tai Chi, mindfulness and similar disciplines, is where we seek to escape from the preoccupations of the mind, ideally into a state of peace and joy.

Reaching this state on a regular basis can be a long journey, but any moment that we can still the mind is a step on that journey. So, what I'm offering to you now is a lying relaxation, or more precisely a pratyāhāra or sense-withdrawal, based simply on awareness of your breath.

Any of the lying rest positions described earlier will be suitable, so long as you have a little space around you into which to move your arms. Maybe you will experience a little of that 'breathfulness' feeling.

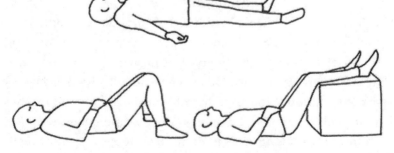

Figure 17. Three possible lying positions for rest

EXERCISE 3.6: The Silent Pause. First, maybe, set a gentle sound to ring on your phone in about 10 minutes (but silence any calls!). Once you are settled in, focus on your breathing. Your breath can be free, all you need to do is to watch your breath going through its natural, relaxed cycle.

Once this too has settled, ask your breath to pause for a moment after every out-breath. If a train of thought arises, stop it in this pause. Even repeat to yourself the word 'Silence'. If you start to feel sleepy, rest the hands on the body. Each time you breathe in, take the backs of your hands out to rest on the floor. Return your hands as you breathe out. You can even add BR>MM to improve your focus. Otherwise, let your breath continue, always turning around smoothly.

When you hear the gentle chime which you have set, don't jump up at once. Take several deep breaths, yawn and stretch, before opening your eyes, getting up slowly and continuing your day.

Another way to maintain your concentration is to keep returning in your mind to a previous peaceful, joyful experience. This was taught to me by Mr AG Mohan, www.svastha.net, who studied breathwork with Krishnamacharya. As he explained to me, these past impressions don't fade with use, if anything they become stronger.

Managing fear

Our teacher, Mr Desikachar, told us he'd found that people were far more nervous about holding their breath out than holding it in. So please congratulate yourself on working through this chapter. Whenever we embark on a new activity, there is always some trepidation. What I've learnt working as a yoga teacher is that people are more anxious, on the whole, about working with their breath than with their bodies. However, your breath is, in a sense, more alive than your body and wants to help you, if you'll let it.

Nonetheless, you may have been experiencing some reasonable fears.

When you started, you were concerned that your breath wasn't working very well. However, you may have wondered if, by asking it to change, you'd experience yet more difficulty. That may have been true to a small extent and that's another reason why I've broken things down into small steps, not because I doubt your ability, but because you and your breath will need time to make small, comfortable adjustments.

Maybe you thought that if people knew you were working with your breath, that they'd pester you with questions about your progress. If you have felt that you've made some, just say that. Or, if you'd rather not talk about it, just tell them it's too early to say. You don't need to say anything, except maybe to encourage others to do some practice with their breath. Whatever reason you may have had for trepidation, you won't have been alone in feeling that way. Maybe speak to a yoga teacher, if you have one, or to a friend who will simply listen and accept.

'...is it not possible for all of us to be in an environment where there is no fear but rather an atmosphere of freedom...? To live is to find out for yourself what is true, and you can only do this where there is freedom...' (Krishnamurti, 1964, p94).

As an aside, I'm aware that there are organisations or practitioners who teach controlled rapid breathing over a long period, a sort of managed hyperventilation, taught under close supervision. I've read that this can bring about an emotional release. When I tried this years ago, I found that my habitual fears and tensions 're-grew' over the following weeks and months spent in my 'normal' home and work environment. My belief, therefore, is that such sudden releases, however well-managed, will need a lot of follow-ups to have any lasting benefit.

It's the same with any breathwork; a study in India with asthma sufferers saw dramatic improvements in the course of a residential program; however, those patients who did not keep up the breathing exercises after leaving the program gradually relapsed.

EXERCISES SUMMARY CHAPTER 3:

3.1 Trial pause between breaths preceded by optional Ū exhale
3.2 Repeated pause between breaths, extending from 2 to 4 seconds or more
3.3 Arm movement and smooth out-breath turn-around
3.4 Exhale > Movement, arm movement in a standing position
3.5 Exhale & Inhale > Movement, arm movement in a standing position
3.6 The Silent Pause in relaxed lying

Step-by-step – 3

The exercises in this chapter were more sophisticated and assumed you'd got used to coordinating breath and movement. Also, that you'd learned to pause after both exhale and inhale to turn your breath around smoothly and to do this even while your arms were still. These techniques are designed to help keep your attention in the exercises, to be mindful – and breathful – and avoid too much mental wandering.

Our next chapter assumes a certain degree of mindfulness, together with a relaxed attitude to allowing your breath to work from within. The above exercises will have prepared you for what comes next; however, they can also be repeated whenever you feel you need more time at this stage.

This can be true, especially, if you are following these exercises to gain relief from asthma or other breathing difficulty.

While you may stand to gain the most from the exercises in this book, you may also face greater challenges.

Above all, be patient with yourself and with your breath. It takes roughly 3 weeks to become proficient in a new technique and about 3 months before it will be ingrained. Please take things one step at a time!

Chapter 4

Open Your Heart

Back when I was a tense and anxious teenager this was reflected in my posture, which had become somewhat closed and stooped. I tried at the time to correct this by pulling my shoulders back. It was 20 years later in 1985 when I started having private lessons with Paul Harvey, https://yogastudies.org, that I began to understand that this tightness could only be fully addressed through recruiting my breath.

One of the most natural and joyful feelings that we can have is the sensation of the in-breath gradually opening space in the body, starting just below the throat, then opening forward of the heart and then a deeper feeling of expansion spreading into the lower ribs and the abdomen, even as far as filling the pelvic bowl, then turning the breath gently around and feeling it being lifted slowly and smoothly up and out again. I think of this as 'heart-first' breathing.

EXERCISE 4.1: Serene upper chest out-lift or heart-first breathing. This is as much an aspiration as an exercise. Place your hands on the upper chest, first three fingers on each hand pointing towards the base of the throat, shoulders relaxed, as in Figure 18. See if you can invite your breath to come in and begin creating space under your fingers before it flows further down. Exhale from your tummy, which by now is beginning to feel normal for you. The degree of physical out-lift on inhaling will be just enough to be felt.

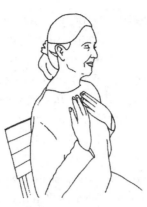

Figure 18. Serene upper chest out-lift by the in-breath, guided by this gesture at the throat

If you didn't feel this, or if this doesn't seem an attractive idea, a note of caution is needed here. The heart area is where we experience love and joy, but also grief and other emotional pain. In these cases, the breath may have learnt ways of avoiding any opening of this area. If you think this may apply to you, then my advice is to seek the guidance of an experienced teacher. The Society of Yoga Practitioners (www.tsyp.yoga), of which I am a founder member, keeps a register of teachers in the UK and nearby countries qualified to guide you through a process of gradual heart opening, based on the approach to be revealed in the first section of this chapter. Other links are given in Chapter 8.

On a more physical level, I was recently monitoring my blood oxygen saturation (%SpO_2) while recovering from Covid-19. The above practice helped consistently to lift my reading by 1-2 per cent. Something I remembered during my recovery is that constant coughing tends to put one into a rather chest-closed posture which can stay in place even after the chest has cleared up and the back and ribs, etc. have recovered. The practices you will learn in this chapter are ones to remember when you are recovering from a chest infection.

Why breathe into your upper chest?

My approach to heart-first breathing began with two questions: (1) Why do many yoga teachers associate breathing into the upper chest with anxiety and stress and (2) why do so many students find that their shoulders lift when they're asked to breathe into the chest first? What I found was that these two questions are closely related and that the same approach would answer them both.

Earlier, we looked at rapid, shallow, anxious breathing, but didn't go into the mechanics. Clearly, shallow breathing means breathing into the upper chest and not much deeper. In order to get enough air in this way, the breath recruits what are known as accessory breathing muscles in the neck and shoulders. These can't help very much, actually. To use them means we are drawing on an emergency response, one the body ought to keep for when it has to cope with an extreme need for air. However, it is a misconception that all breathing into the upper chest necessarily falls into this anxious, emergency category.

A few years ago, when I'd been teaching people to start their in-breaths in their chests for many years, I still hadn't figured how to help my students do this without lifting their shoulders. They still looked stressed, so I had to keep looking for a way for them to open the heart area to the in-breath that wasn't, or didn't look, anxious.

My 'light bulb moment' came when I suggested to one of my private students that she ask her breath to come in and create space 'forward of her heart'. These words; the idea, the feeling, the impression of space being created forward of the heart was, and is, vital. I was emulating the way that Mr Desikachar taught us to use our imagination, to wish for what we sought to experience, using what he called a 'bhāvana' (long first ā as in 'calm'). The words that my student used at the time to describe this feeling was 'magic, Michael, that's magic!'

Creating space

Bhāvana, the creation of an imaginative impression, is a common idea in yoga and one which our teacher, Mr Desikachar, was right to emphasise. At the root of this Sanskrit word is the idea of bringing something into being. If we can focus and imagine in a certain way, we can experience something that was always a possibility, but one of which we were unaware. That's why bhāvana can sometimes feel like magic.

EXERCISE 4.2: Feeling your in-breath forward of your heart. If you feel ready to try this, it's very simple. Place your hands comfortably over your heart and simply ask your breath, each time it comes in, to create a little space forward of your heart. Breathe out slowly this time as learnt previously. Imagine and wish to feel this space. It's important to avoid any sense that you're forcing your breath to do this, especially if you have suffered from asthma. The feeling must be that your breath is doing it all, albeit at your request. It doesn't matter if the feeling of opening forward is hesitant and slight; with daily practice it can only get stronger. You are drawing on the patience which you cultivated in chapters 1-3.

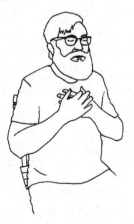

Figure 19. Bhāvana of asking your in-breath to create space
forward of your heart

We asked, in the previous section, if chest breathing need always reflect anxiety. You can discover, through your own experience, that this isn't so and then the way ahead will be open. If you can allow your breath to do the work in a gentle passive way, you will begin to cut the ground from underneath any tendency to anxious breathing. You will be able to sense and feel your breath entering and flowing in down through the body in the direction of its own natural flow and the reverse on your out-breath, flowing up and out through your body. You will begin to experience 'breathfulness' without making any outward movement. Don't, however, try this exercise while waiting at traffic lights, or for more than a minute or two when at work, you might get lost in it!

Can we actually feel the flow of the breath under our breastbones? From a short conversation with Dr Stephen Porges at the Yoga Therapy Conference in Amsterdam, April 2019, I believe that we can gradually increase our conscious awareness of this subtle inner sensation.

More prosaically, this exercise can help release any trapped wind in the stomach or relieve slight nausea. If this is the case, ask your breath to start coming in forward of the heart but only descend, each time, as far as is comfortable.

Please remember that we are looking for millimetre movements which can only be made by your breath working from within and being guided by feeling and imagination (bhāvana). Your breath is the most powerful force at your disposal; however, it's not one you should try to command; you must work with it in a spirit of cooperation. As these micro-movements develop with daily practice, they can bring about profound and lasting improvements in your upper body posture.

EXERCISE 4.3: Lifting your hands off your heart as you feel your breath start to come in. To build on this impression, this 'bhāvana', you can bring the lifting and lowering of the arms into play. Consistently with the idea of BR>MM from Exercise 3.5, you can begin by asking the breath to create a little space forward of your heart. As you feel your breath wanting to go down deeper, lift your arms up and out in an expansive, opening gesture. Pause your arms in a lifted position, shoulders relaxed, while you check that your breath has entered fully. Allow it to gently turn around. As your breath is flowing out, slowly return your hands to your heart and wait for the next breath to be ready.

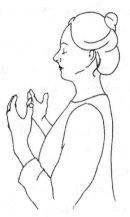

Figure 20. As Figure 19, but now, as your breath starts to come in, it seems to lift your hands off your heart

Relaxing your neck and shoulders

Now you've discovered that you have a possible solution, an alternative, to anxious upper chest breathing, then it ought to help those poor overworked accessory muscles in the neck and shoulders to relax. Let's try it and find out.

EXERCISE 4.4: Pause to release your shoulders. The first way you're going to do this is to repeat the exercise in the last section, but adding a slight pause between breaths. In that pause, focus on the *idea* of your shoulders relaxing, dropping, letting-go. Do not try to force your shoulders down; invite them to simply let go. Repeat this exercise at least 6 times, which will give you 6 opportunities for something to happen. In a way, you're just checking your shoulders each time to say to them 'let go'.

Compared to learning to let go of tension in the shoulders, finding a way to lessen tension in the neck can require us to be more resourceful. For a start, we are going to need a whole long, smooth exhale to work on this. Added to that, we will have to bring in another bhāvana or imaginative impression.

EXERCISE 4.5: Wishing for Space (Figure 21). Place your hands comfortably on your chest, this time a little above the heart, with your first two fingers pointing up towards your throat. Invite your breath in, forward of the heart, as before. When the breath has filled completely, turn it round gently, starting from low down. As your breath flows out, start to imagine, to create a new, additional bhāvana.

This bhāvana is of a *wish* to feel some space at the base of your throat spreading down your breastbone as you inhale. Combined with this is a feeling of the back of your head lifting and your shoulders continuing to soften away from a point at the base of your neck. Continue with your breathing cycle and as you breathe in, you may find the neck and shoulders are relaxing even more.

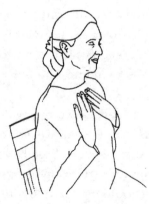

Figure 21. A gesture to bring attention to the base of your throat, and with your in-breath a wish to create space there

You have now successfully turned upper chest breathing from having an association with tension to being a source of relaxation. As you keep up your requests for space both front and back, the feeling of passive letting-go will build. You may feel that your breastbone is lifting towards your chin, which may drop a little as your neck relaxes. Avoid any tendency to hurry this process. Only continue as long as it feels relaxing. It's important to *let your breath do all the work*.

EXERCISE 4.6: Adding a gentle backward arm drop standing (Figure 22). Once this feeling, that you're opening space from the throat to the heart as you start to breathe in, is established, see if you can keep that feeling while holding your clasped hands loosely behind your back. Please do not tense your shoulders back, just ask them to drop backward, but do straighten your arms very gently as you inhale. Let your in-breath do the work of opening, then remember to let it continue in and down. Breathe out slowly, relaxing your arms. Like the previous exercises, this is very passive, you're still asking your breath to do most of the work.

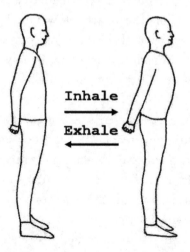

Figure 22. Backward arm drop, maintaining the sense of space across the top of the chest and at the back of the neck

As with the use of sound with the abdominal exhalation (see Chapter 2 under 'Simple Sounds'), releasing in the heart area can sometimes allow tears to arise. Please look again at the advice in Chapter 2. But tears are most likely to happen if you feel safe and have, either to hand or nearby, someone to whom you can talk about these feelings.

When you take a mental step back and let your breath do the work, that is a step towards a state of non-doing, where all conscious effort has been set aside. In this state, you feel that your breath and everything else is simply going along naturally and you experience this joyful, peaceful state of breathfulness. This is why the ancient yogis emphasised patience, gentleness, subtlety, lack of any hurry. These are qualities we can work on until a peaceful, mindful awareness of breathing simply falls into place.

The 'Magic' breath

While 'magic' is what my student first called it, I've been using the term 'heart-first' breath. Mr Desikachar used to teach an exercise which incorporated this; he called it the 'caring breath' because it centred on the heart. However, he advised those suffering from asthma or back pain to approach this exercise cautiously. Like many things in yoga, it may help greatly, so long as one is not in a hurry to get results.

EXERCISE 4.7: Mr Desikachar's 'Caring Breath'. This can be done standing with your feet a little apart or, as described here, sitting upright with space to sweep your arms out to each side. Place your hands over your heart, right hand on top. We are going to use bhāvana again, this time of your breath creating space under your left, resting, hand.

When your breath wants to come in, stretch your right hand smoothly out to the side at shoulder level. Feel your breath enter under your left hand. Start to breathe out from below and slowly return your right hand. Repeat, this time opening your left hand out to your left. Let your body relax and feel some movement right down into your seat. Also, turn your head the same way as you move each hand. But never swing your arm rapidly so it comes to a sudden stop, please work smoothly.

I think that, without putting it in so many words, Mr Desikachar was giving people this exercise to ease and stretch the muscle and fascia across their chests; tightness in these can be a limiting factor in reopening this area.

However, as a scientist writing this book and studying the mechanisms of breathing, I really wanted to know, physically, what this 'heart first' or 'caring breath' consisted of. I have to thank Patrick McKeown for a reference in his more recent and much larger book 'The Breathing Cure' (McKeown, 2021, p173) to a little-known set of muscles each side of the breastbone, the parasternal intercostal muscles. I shall refer to them from now on as just the 'parasternals'. As shown in Figure 23, these muscles fill the spaces between your six upper ribs, where these ribs change from bone to softer cartilage and meet your breastbone in front.

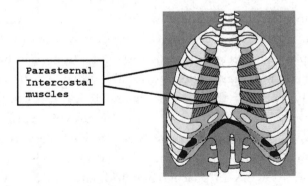

Figure 23. Where to locate your parasternals. They are shown here as shaded and cross-hatched areas filling the spaces between your soft ribs each side of your breastbone (sternum). The diaphragm is shown in its contracted, breath-in position

The function of your parasternals in relaxed, downflow breathing is to keep the front of your chest open. At the back you have your fairly stiff, supporting upper spine. Holding the sides of your chest open are your hoop-shaped ribs, like the arches in a building. So as your diaphragm descends and creates negative pressure in your chest, in order to draw air into your lungs, the back and sides of your ribcage remain firm. But the front of your chest is both softer and flatter; if it were not for this, chest compressions in emergency resuscitation would be impossible!

Now we can see that, if it were not for your parasternals engaging to steady this area, the suction created in your chest, as you breathe in, would pull your breastbone inwards, reducing the effectiveness of your diaphragm. Therefore, as soon as you need to inhale, your parasternals hold the front of your chest open so that your diaphragm can work to full effect. As your diaphragm relaxes on your exhalation, so can your parasternals, until your next breath is needed. This account of their operation is based on the work of Prof André De Troyer of the Brussels School of Medicine (De Troyer, 1991).

This important role of the parasternals in relaxed quiet breathing, in what I call 'downflow' inhaling, is very little known. In relaxed breathing, all the parasternals do is hold the upper chest steady. If you press your fingers in between your third and fourth ribs and inhale with your diaphragm, you may feel your third parasternals engage, but produce no movement. In practice, it's not easy to feel your parasternals working; you'd have to press your fingers very firmly in between your ribs, which could be painful. So just let your parasternals work in peace! Their hidden nature is why the parasternals have been so overlooked and the role of the upper chest in relaxed breathing so widely ignored. The parasternals are of especial importance in our earliest years when the chest wall is very soft.

Your parasternals are purely breathing muscles and have no other role. While your diaphragm can be made to work, in a way, by consciously expanding your lower ribs without inhaling, you cannot contract your parasternals independently of your in-breath. So, apart from the more subjective, calming effect of the 'heart-first' or 'caring' breath, learning to activate your parasternals to create a tiny outward movement of your breastbone gives important confirmation that your parasternals are ready to assist with your every relaxed, quiet, conscious or unconscious breath.

In experiments reported by Gandevia et al (2006), it was found that activity in the parasternals 'sometimes preceded inspiratory airflow'. This confirmation is important for all of us who follow Mr Desikachar, since he always taught us to focus in that same area at the start of each in-breath. His father, Srī Krishnamacharya, would undoubtedly have known this and everything else about the breath from the inside out, without the benefit of modern physiology.

Patrick McKeown (2021, p176) also draws attention to research at South Korea's Konyang University (Kang et al, 2018), which showed that learning diaphragmatic (i.e., downflow) breathing improves the mobility of the sternum (breastbone), providing further evidence of the synergy between the parasternal area and the diaphragm in functional breathing. On the same page, McKeown argues that bracing the core muscles without functional involvement of the diaphragm can be counter-productive when it comes to countering back pain. Again, we must work with the breath!

Now we must consider our lower ribs. In relaxed breathing, intra-abdominal pressure opens our lower ribs passively; however, these ribs need to be freely moving for this to happen. While we can consciously expand our lower ribs, independently of our breath, working *with* our breath is always the best course of action.

Expanding your lower ribs

For a few years, I used to present Saturday morning seminars, a few times a year, at the studio of a teacher whom I trained about 10 years ago. One Saturday, at the break after the first warm-up practice of movement and breathing, a man came up to me and said, 'Michael, I didn't know I could breathe so much!' So, what had I been teaching? It was actually quite simple.

Let's do some limbering first. I learnt this exercise from Dr N Chandrasekharan (https://yogavaidyasala.net) (he likes to be called, simply, Dr NC). NC is a medical doctor who also trained in Ayurveda – traditional Indian medicine – and furthermore trained as a yoga therapist with Mr Desikachar. Having taught for a while at Mr Desikachar's institute, the Krishnamacharya Yoga Mandiram (KYM) in Chennai, Dr NC is now one of the world's leading trainers of yoga therapists.

EXERCISE 4.8: Dr NC's upright twist (Figure 24). You'll again need space to sweep your arms out to both sides and also a surface, such as a yoga mat, with enough grip that you can place your feet securely, about your arm's length apart, without any tendency to slide. Place your hands just above your navel, one hand on top. We are going to use bhāvana again, this time of your breath creating space under your hands.

When your breath wants to come in against your underneath hand, slide it out and stretch it out smoothly round to the side while completing your in-breath. Allow a gentle twist to occur from head to foot. Also, turn your head the same way as you are turning in the body. But never swing your arm so it comes to a sudden stop. Start to breathe out from below, slowly returning your hand as you come out of the twist.

As in Exercise 2.3, avoid a 'ballistic stretch' which, as well as causing strain where your ribs join your spine, can stress your knees.

Repeat to your other side, sliding your opposite hand out and round to lead you into a smooth turning movement. Relax and feel some movement right down into your feet. Return your hand, breathing out from below. Repeat to the first side and so on until you've completed six stretches in total. Once you have breath and movement coordinated, you can focus on the bhāvana of each in-breath creating space under your hand. This exercise can be repeated once a day, most days.

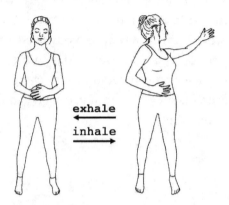

Figure 24. Dr NC's upright opening twist, standing

EXERCISE 4.9: Expanding your ribcage. Once you are confident with Exercise 4.8, try sliding your hand on each side as far round onto your side ribs as comfortable. Now, simply ask your in-breath to lift your ribs outwards to both sides. You may feel a need to yawn; let this happen. You may feel more lifting of your ribs on one side; this is often the case. For instance, we can habitually hold more tension, more tightness on one side of the body.

EXERCISE 4.10: 'Banana' Pose. The gentlest way I have found to work on this tightness is in a certain lying position (see Figure 25) also taught to me by Dr NC. Again, you will need space to spread your arms out to both sides. In this position, stretch your legs out straight (Note: If there is tenderness or weakness in your lower back, try this first with your knees bent and your feet flat on your mat.).

Then, in very small steps, walk your heels along the floor away from the tighter side of your ribs. Only walk the heels as far as you can without the hips starting to tilt. Then relax and ask your in-breath each time to ease the tighter side a little more open. It may help to slide the hand on that side a little higher on each in-breath.

After 6 breaths, breathing deeply and freely, walk your heels over to the other side. Compare, now, what 6 breaths feel like on the easier side. Then slowly walk your heels back across the centre line to repeat the exercise on the first side. After this, walk your heels back to centre and draw the feet up towards you. Rest your hands on your tummy and take at least 6 breaths of gentle abdominal breathing.

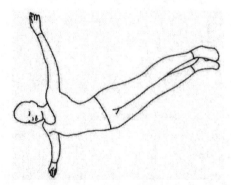

Figure 25. 'Banana' Lying Pose, intended to gently open one flank to invite the breath to ease out some further opening

When I was working as an experimental physicist on a particular project in the mid-late 1980s, there was a very minor risk of exposure to a toxic dust. Every year, my breathing capacity (FVC) and flow (FEV1) were being measured to check for any early signs of a problem. Also, I was at an age (35-40) when, according to the statistics, my FVC and FEV1 would start to decline. However, over the years I was being tested, these same measurements gradually increased and remained the same when I was tested again, as part of the UK Biobank study, nearly 20 years later. An analysis (Schünemann et al, 2000) of the Buffalo Health Study, which followed the health of over 1000 residents of Buffalo, NY for 29 years, showed a direct relationship between maintaining FEV1 and longevity.

In summary

Most upper chest breathing isn't helpful and may be positively dysfunctional. In contrast, the *functional* contribution to breathing from the upper chest of which you are now aware, while little-known, is an important feature of our natural 'quiet' breathing cycle. A slight initial contribution to each inhalation from the upper chest is not only allowable, but natural.

Focusing on this contribution, consciously, puts us in a frame of mind to follow the path of our breath as it flows inwards and, to repeat again the words of Mr Desikachar, 'acutely sense and feel the movement of the breath within'. With my fellow yoga teachers in mind, I plan to return to this functional upper chest breathing in a later volume, when I shall have a chance to discuss the yoga technique known as Bandha.

EXERCISES SUMMARY CHAPTER 4:
4.1 Serene upper chest out-lift
4.2 Asking your in-breath to create space forward of your heart
4.3 Lifting your hands off your heart
4.4 Pause to release the shoulders
4.5 Wishing for Space
4.6 Adding a gentle backward arm stretch
4.7 Mr Desikachar's 'Caring Breath'
4.8 Dr NC's upright twist
4.9 Expanding your ribcage
4.10 'Banana' Pose

Step-by-step – 4

The exercises in this chapter will have taken you deeper into 'sensing the movement of the breath within', as Mr Desikachar put it. How did it feel to be working at this level of sophistication? Is the idea of 'breathfulness' becoming more real for you and, in focusing more on your ribs, did you keep contact with your core muscles? If so, you have now learnt something that you can apply whenever you have a need. As one of my students put it:

> I like the breathing you do in your classes because you can bring that breathing that you've learnt into play wherever you are.
>
> Jackie

This chapter, as well as focusing on the heart, has also been the heart of this book. My next chapter returns to the idea of being comfortable with using your core muscles, both with gently engaging them and with letting-go with them, if gravity will do their work instead.

Addendum: finger sweeping

This exercise doesn't contribute to relearning your breathing cycle, but was mentioned earlier by one of my students, Patricia. She'd taught her mother the ancient yoga practice of Kara Nyāsa and I promised to describe this for you. This practice belongs with this chapter because it can help to induce a subtle heart-opening feeling.

Sitting comfortably, place the tip of each forefinger on the inside base of each thumb. Exhale slowly. As your breath comes in, slide your fingers to the tips of your thumbs. As you breathe out, sweep your thumb again from base to tip, this time along the outside. Flick your thumbs off your fingers.

Pause your breath a moment to bring the tip of each thumb to the inside base of each forefinger. As you inhale, sweep your thumbs up your fingers; as you exhale, sweep your thumbs over the tops of your forefingers, from base to tip. Flick your fingers off your thumbs. Repeat for your second, third and little fingers.

Finally, breathing in, sweep the insides of your forearms and out to your fingers with the palms of your hands. As you breathe out, with your palms, quickly sweep the backs of both arms and hands. Without hesitation, loosely clench both fists and then flick all your fingers forwards. Repeat the whole exercise 3 times. You can think about this as an extension of the heart-first breath, so long as this comes naturally.

There are a number of versions of Kara Nyāsa, but this is the one taught to me by Mr Desikachar. This was when I asked him for something for my late father-in-law, who suffered from Parkinson's Disease. This disabling condition can be most keenly felt by sufferers once it affects the hands, the use of our hands being so much taken for granted. My teacher's aim was to help my father-in-law keep the use of his hands as long as possible.

Chapter 5

Hips above Heart

When I was training as a yoga therapist with Paul Harvey, from 1987 to 1990, he told us that half of yoga is simply looking after yourself.

If you see pictures of yogis and their students either standing on their heads or in other upside-down poses, this is only one piece of the massive jigsaw puzzle which is yoga. I venture that very few people fully understand why these inversions are done, even if they practise inversions themselves, for the sake of their calming effect. When, in everyday life, do we even slightly invert our bodies, take our hips above our hearts, our hearts above our heads? Even if we are somewhat 'bendy', this might only happen for a moment, when we stoop to pick something up off the floor.

When we do stay, even for a short while, with our hips just a short distance above our hearts, we are doing something out of the ordinary. We are going to feel some unusual effects and certainly we don't need to start with headstands.

Appreciate your diaphragm

As soon as you assume an even slightly inverted position, you will notice an effect on your breath.

EXERCISE 5.1: Supported mild elevation (Figure 26). If you want a very easy way to begin, prepare yourself to rest on your back with about 4 inches (10 cm) of support under your hips and with your lower legs and feet supported on the seat of a chair. A thinner support under the head may benefit your neck. If you have yoga blocks, two full thickness ones under your hips will do, if not, you can improvise with some large, thick books and a thin cushion on top.

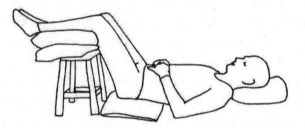

Figure 26. Supported lying, hips and legs raised

In this position, you'll be returning to the abdominal breathing you learnt at the end of Chapter 1. However, now you'll find that more effort is needed to lift your breath in from your heart towards your hips. Also, you'll need to learn how to let your breath out slowly, since there's now more of a positive drive behind it.

Let's look at what's actually doing that work for you and your breath. As described at the end of Chapter 1, your respiratory diaphragm divides your body into upper and lower spaces and its job is to contract and flatten towards your abdomen when your breath comes in, assisted by the expansion of your lower ribs. This creates more space for air to enter your upper body, while (in standing or sitting) pushing down on your lower organs.

When you have your hips above your heart, your diaphragm has to work harder, since more of the weight of your abdominal organs rests on it, when compared to lying flat. Consider, if you can feel an effect even with your hips just 4 inches (10 cm) above your heart, what's a headstand going to feel like? In a follow-up to this book, I will describe how there's no point in attempting a headstand unless and until you can breathe deeply once you're there.

Moving the piston

EXERCISE 5.2: Lying, passive slight inversion: Assume the same comfortable supported lying position as in Exercise 5.1, legs above the hips, hips above the heart. Rest your hands on your belly. Inhale slowly, feeling your diaphragm push your abdomen up and away to create more space for your lungs. Let your breath turn around smoothly and watch as, smoothly and progressively, your diaphragm slowly relaxes to allow your breath to flow evenly. Repeat this exercise for up to 10 more breaths, feeling that there's something like a piston in your body (Figure 27), easing your breath in and up and easing it back out and down again.

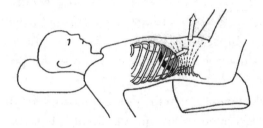

Figure 27. Piston action of the diaphragm (darker shaded area inside the ribs) to lift the abdominal wall in slightly raised lying

If you do wish to go on to deeper, more demanding, inversions, this will be the foundation of your practice. However, while we're here at this first easy stage, let's look at the initial benefits:

- By repeated practice, for up to 12 breaths at a time in this position, you will be strengthening your diaphragm to work in its optimal mode.
- You will be giving your heart a chance to feel some assistance, since every time you breathe in extra blood will be returned to the heart, due to the pressure on the abdominal organs from the diaphragm.

- Your diaphragm will be learning to work smoothly, despite the slight inversion, both on inhale and exhale.
- Yoga inversions can have a calming effect, which you may feel even in this initial position.

As always, please allow your breath to work gently and smoothly. As soon as we try to force or hurry the breath to do something, there is the danger of creating a resistance, or of causing ill-effects. This patient manner of daily practice will do more to strengthen your diaphragm than even high-intensity athletics. Apparently, such activities can fatigue the diaphragm, resulting in breathlessness, without improving its strength (Amman, 2012). Maybe that's what happened to my student on her uphill bike-ride with her grandchildren. Certainly, we can expect that using one's diaphragm in a less than optimal way will more readily cause it to fatigue.

Deeper letting-go

Another key beneficial effect of inverting the body, even a little, is the release that can be experienced in the abdominal area. This sort of release is especially valuable for anyone with a more sedentary lifestyle, in which the abdominal organs see very little relative movement or shift of weight.

In order to complete the previous two exercises, you will have used your back and thigh muscles to lift your hips off your mat to place a block or cushion underneath. If you found that comfortable, we can make this into an exercise in itself.

EXERCISE 5.3: Lying, active semi-inversion: You will need to start in a lying position with your feet drawn up close to you so the knees are raised. Both feet and knees need to be about hip-width apart. Relax your arms along by your sides, palms down.

Important, REMOVE any support from under your head unless (exceptionally) your teacher says this is okay.

Very importantly, face directly upwards throughout the exercise and NEVER turn your head to look to one side, while your hips are raised. Doing so could strain your neck.

Take a breath or two to relax into your initial resting position. When your breath next wants to come in, put some weight into your feet and feel your hips lift off the mat. Complete your in-breath with your hips raised, start to breathe out and, on your long out-breath, lower your hips smoothly. Practise these lifts 5 more times, so long as it's comfortable.

NEVER continue if there is pain or anything more than the mild discomfort that can arise from trying something unfamiliar.

Rest, and as you breathe in lift your feet off the mat and bring your hands to your knees and your knees to your hands. Breathe out and relax into the second (Apānāsana) position in Figure 28, breathing freely, letting your body soften. It's okay now to pop a thin cushion under your head. If bringing in both knees at once isn't comfortable, bring in one knee to relax for a few breaths and then the same with the other.

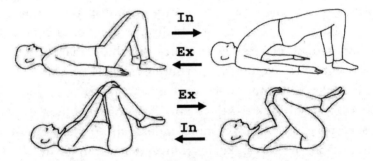

Figure 28. Dvī Pāda Pītham (Half Bridge) & Apānāsana

If you've happily completed this exercise, you can use this movement to experience more abdominal release.

EXERCISE 5.4: Letting your abdomen sink: Return your feet to your mat, close to your body, hip-width apart as before, no head support. Looking straight up, breathe in and lift your hips. Before you lower your hips, start to let your breath go, letting your stomach sink in towards your spine. Then continue your out-breath, lowering the hips to the mat. Take a free breath, then repeat. Continue to repeat up to four more times, taking one free breath between lifts.

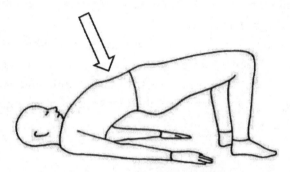

Figure 29. Letting-go of the abdomen in Dvī Pāda Pītham (Half Bridge)

You may find that you can feel the effect of your in-breath up into the pelvic bowl and feel a release there as you start to exhale.

Upright directional breathing

Have you noticed that we're working towards something here, that a direction is appearing both in your in-breath and in your out-breath? In parallel with the natural direction of flow of air in and down, followed by up and back out again, you've developed a sense of your breath – and feelings associated with it – descending as you breathe in and ascending as you breathe out. Mr Desikachar referred to this as 'directional breathing'. You don't have to be lying on your back or lifting your hips off the mat to experience this. Once this pattern has been established, you can contact it in any position, including an upright seated position.

EXERCISE 5.5: Upright Directional Breathing (Figure 30): Sitting comfortably, place one hand on your heart and the other on your tummy. Breathe out slowly and then invite your breath to come in progressively as it's done before, lifting first forward of your heart, and then feeling the tummy expand. Let your breath turn around smoothly, starting your out-breath by lifting your tummy in. Your chest will naturally relax, ready to receive your next in-breath.

Stay with this practice for about 12 breaths to help it become established. Then sit quietly for a minute or two observing the free breath. If at any point you start to feel light-headed, pause and wait for the need to breathe in to become stronger before continuing.

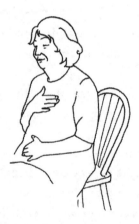

Figure 30. Upright comfortable sitting with one hand on the heart and the other on the tummy

What you and your breath have re-established here is the full coordination of your entire apparatus of natural breathing, something you may have been missing since childhood. This new pattern, regularly practised, will in time resume its natural place in your life. When you notice your relaxed, unconscious breathing, the lift that occurs forward of your heart will be almost imperceptible and your breath will be mostly felt lower down. You will feel relaxed with just a touch of necessary alertness. Like a wave approaching the coast, the in-breath starts as a tiny lift in the upper chest, gradually swells, is felt most fully in the tummy and finally washes out towards the hips. After a very light initial lift from below, your out-breath is a slow, relaxing letting-go.

You don't need to focus on this directional breathing 24/7. One of its aims is to gradually open a heart area that may have become closed in the course of life. For me, this closure happened in my early teens. I still practise this myself, now and then, so long as I have a quiet place to focus, to open my heart area and relax my neck and shoulders. Otherwise, I simply breathe softly through my nose and let my breath decide how best to work.

Full inversion?

It's hard to leave off writing about inversions without a word about the full inversions, such as headstands and shoulder stands, that are so often associated with yoga. A telling personal story has been shared by Dr Timothy McCall (McCall, 2007, p.90). He reports on a visit he made to the KYM:

> The teacher at the KYM said headstand and the other āsana they wanted me to stop could be contributing to my problems by compressing my neck and spine, something I had figured out on my own. To address the problem, they recommended a series of gentle backbends and other poses designed to open my chest. A few days later…it occurred to me that for the first time in a month my arm hadn't gone numb all day.

The symptom that Dr McCall is describing here is of thoracic outlet syndrome, in which the upper chest becomes so closed that the nerves to the arms can become compressed. Now it's clear why we covered heart-first, heart-opening breathwork and movements in the previous chapter, before taking even a cautious look at inversions. Later on the same page, McCall later quotes Krishnamacharya's description of headstand as 'The king of the asanas', but I was unwise to attempt it before I'd had a couple of years' training with Paul Harvey, similar to that described by McCall.

Something you may read in older books on yoga is that inversions increase the supply of oxygen to the brain. This idea is completely mistaken! As Professor Kim Parker (Dept. Bioengineering, Imperial College) explained in the course of our many very helpful discussions on the potential effects of yoga inversions, the supply of oxygen to every cell in the brain is very carefully regulated; even a little too much oxygen is more dangerous than not quite enough. As my own research has shown, blood flow to the brain is largely protected against the effects of postural changes (Hutchinson, 2011). The way to improve oxygenation of the brain, if feeling faint, is to breathe into your lower lungs and breathe out slowly with a little resistance in your nose or throat. Your circulatory system will then be able to deliver the optimum amount of oxygen to each part of your brain. Rapid breathing, on the other hand, can actually reduce oxygen availability.

Breath and posture

It's time now to summarise how correct breathing and correct posture support each other. People notice that I can sit upright for an hour with no apparent effort. This is because of the way that I breathe, the way that I've been teaching you. Given time and daily practice, asking your in-breath to keep your heart area open straightens your upper back, without any effort from you. It also helps your neck and shoulders to be more relaxed. Activating your core muscles to gently engage as you breathe out keeps up a gentle intra-abdominal pressure that supports your lower back in an easy way. It also helps the return of blood to your heart. And finally, this open, upright but relaxed posture allows your breath optimum access to your lungs. This is how Mr Desikachar told us to improve our breathing and posture, 30 years ago:

'Directional breathing,' he emphasised, 'has an effect on the spine. The ancients said to inhale from chest to abdomen, it is like an offering...Do not insist upon it for everyone and take care of those with asthma or back pain.' (Desikachar, 1992)

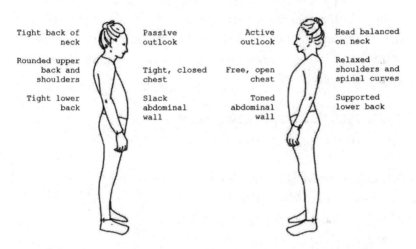

Tight back of neck | Passive outlook | Active outlook | Head balanced on neck
Rounded upper back and shoulders | Tight, closed chest | Free, open chest | Relaxed shoulders and spinal curves
Tight lower back | Slack abdominal wall | Toned abdominal wall | Supported lower back

Figure 31. Contrasting the posture that can result from neglecting the breath, a posture which is both slack and tight, with the firm, relaxed posture that correct work with the breath can maintain. The shoulders aren't pulled back, but fall back naturally once the chest is open

As Figure 31 shows, before learning to work with your breath, you may have been tending towards a chest in-drop and an abdomen out-drop. With time, age and neglect, the chest can become tight and the abdomen slack. With regular patient practice, befriending our breath, we can start to have the opposite effects, a slight chest out-lift and a corresponding abdomen in-lift on every breath you take.

This won't require any continuous conscious effort from you. A relaxed, upright posture and a healthy breathing cycle go hand-in-hand. However, if you notice anytime that your posture isn't ideal, you may just find it helpful to repeat Exercise 5.5.

With an improved breathing cycle, tension in your neck will be reduced or eliminated and headaches resulting from the way that this tension can spread into your jaw, face and scalp will become less frequent. There may even be a slight further opening of your upper air passages, allowing freer nasal breathing.

It's worth noting here that a perfect body is not a requirement for you to engage with yoga. Paul Harvey once told us that some of the most revered ancient yogis had to live with significant physical disabilities.

EXERCISES SUMMARY CHAPTER 5:
5.1: Supported mild elevation.
5.2: Lying, passive slight inversion.
5.3: Lying, active semi-inversion
5.4: Letting your abdomen sink
5.5: Directional Breathing

Step-by-step – 5

It would be hard to practise the exercises in this chapter without 'sensing the movement of the breath within', since your diaphragm will have had to work in quite an obvious way. These exercises will have given you a stronger impression of natural heart to hips inhalation and the corresponding natural outflow from hips to heart under control. Our next chapter returns to the idea of bringing some mental focus into your work with your breath, in ways that are calming in themselves.

It is appropriate at this point to acknowledge the yogi and scientist Swami Kuvalayānanda, who founded the Lonavla Institute for the scientific study of physical yoga in 1924. In his chapter on Ujjāyī (1966), and possibly in earlier editions of 'Prāṇāyāma', he described the correct cycle of directional breathing, based on studies with his guru and on scientific investigation. It's a shame that more attention hasn't been paid to Kuvalayānanda's work in the last 55 years.

Chapter 6

Counting Slowly...

On a weekend break during our studies at the KYM in July 2009, a group of us took a break from the 35°C heat of Chennai in favour of a dip in the ocean at Mahabalipuram. I was, as I thought, happily swimming through the gentle waves as they rolled in. Starting to tire, I looked round and saw the beach was a long way away, with tiny figures of people I could hardly make out, much less cry to for help. I am not a strong swimmer and can only manage a mediocre breast stroke for a few lengths of the pool. But my only thought was to keep going for the shore, keep my feet up and, above all, keep breathing. My breath kept me calm, my breath kept me going. After a long time just keeping going, while the waves blocked my view of the shore, my feet finally touched the sand. So, if you ever feel you're in too deep, trust your breath to see you through.

At the end of the last chapter, I referred to Prāṇāyāma (structured breathing) as one part of a yoga practice. Disordered breathing, that is breathing that is shallow, irregular, rapid, habitually taken through the mouth has always been seen in yoga as dysfunctional, as associated with some kind of distress and possibly part of a vicious cycle that includes a poor mental outlook and even physical disturbance.

Recent medical research has confirmed this view, associating this disturbed or dysfunctional breathing with chronic over-activation of the sympathetic nervous system (SNS). The SNS has its role to play in responding to the challenges that we face in life. However, if we can never 'wind down' our SNS, this constant disturbance leads to indigestion, insomnia, eventual exhaustion and many other possible 'flare-ups' and ailments.

In response, Brown and Gerbarg (2012, p12) describe what their fellow-researchers have termed 'coherent' breathing. What they mean by that is breathing that follows a certain pattern in time, so you breathe in for 4 or 5 seconds and breathe out for 6 seconds and you keep that up for a few minutes. This timed, ratio breathing isn't new; we were taught a version of it when I started my teacher-training in 1983.

However, what wasn't known then was the way in which this structured breathing stimulates the parasympathetic nervous system (PNS).

The PNS, which exists in all mammals, is what enables us to let down our guard when we perceive that we're in a safe situation. When active, it promotes not only healthy digestion and sleep, but also relaxed social interaction. Researchers are now able to monitor the way in which something called 'heart-rate variability' (HRV) responds to structured breathing exercises. The importance of this is that while HRV is easily measured by monitoring your heart-rate, it is also a direct measure of our degree of PNS activation. We can now directly measure the 'relaxation response' first identified by Benson, Beary and Carol (Benson et al, 1974) and see that our breathing exercises are indeed working to help us relax at a deep level.

Ratio breathing

Having been taught breathing ratios as part of my teacher-training in the 1980s, I have continued a daily practice with these ratios for 38 years. On a day-to-day level these exercises, which I started doing in the early evening after work (I was still working full-time as a scientist), would help me to relax – a bit like a dry martini, but healthier in the long-run.

When I'd been practising this for a few years, I was working quietly in my office one day when one of the senior men in the department stormed in. He'd read a paper I'd written and was at 10,000 feet and still climbing! I found myself standing up from behind my desk and continuing to breathe smoothly and deeply while he yelled at me. I was then able to explain, calmly and convincingly, what I'd written. It was like, for the first time, head and heart were working together. Most surprisingly, this senior man, a figure feared by many in the department, then apologised for his outburst. I'd never heard him apologise like that to anyone before – or since.

Please remember, before this happened, I'd been practising ratio breathing daily for 2 or 3 years. With deeper effects like this, there are no rapid results. But please persist, since daily practice with your breath, as you may already have found, helps to keep you sane. As one of my students who's had a very stressful 2 years recently said:

> I brush my teeth every morning to stop my teeth from falling out; I work with my breath every morning to stop my brain from falling out.
>
> Jane

Ratio technique

When we learnt ratio breathing, we were taught to think of each breath as having, potentially, four parts – inhale, pause, exhale, pause – and to write this shorthand in seconds, for example, 4.0.8.0., which written longhand means inhale for 4 seconds, zero pause, exhale for 8 seconds, zero pause, then repeat the same cycle. So why not try this now?

You will need to assume your personal version of a comfortable, upright seated position (I use the acronym 'CUSP'). Up until now, I've assumed that your CUSP will consist of simply sitting on an upright chair, with a cushion behind your lower back, if needed. However, some of you may already have a comfortable floor-sitting pose. In all cases, please ensure that your hips are a little above your knees. This arrangement will help keep your lower back well-aligned and comfortable. By the way, the idea of being in your CUSP also implies that you're in a space with no distractions, or at least none that aren't easy for you to ignore.

EXERCISE 6.1: Ratio Breathing. Set a metronome (there may be an app available for your phone) or simply a small analogue clock with an audible tick where you can hear it. Settle into your CUSP. Close your eyes, place your hands on your heart and invite your breath inward to open first under your hands and then further down. After 4 seconds, start to lift your breath very slowly up and out from below, taking about 8 seconds. Take the next 5 breaths in the same way continuously.

Only if this 4.0.8.0. ratio is really comfortable add a 2-second pause after breathing out and continue for another 6 breaths. If still comfortable, go on until you've completed another 6 breaths with this ratio. Then stay for 6 breaths with an easier ratio, such as 4.0.4.0., i.e., 4 seconds in, 4 seconds out.

One advantage of ratio breathing is that you can set aside a fixed time for it, say 10 minutes in your busy day and, once you're in it, you don't need to worry about the time. Once you've set your ratio and planned your number of breaths, you've fixed the time your practice will take and you can relax into it, into the present moment and take a break from worrying about time, just counting your breaths.

PANS

Repeating again a quote from Mr Desikachar, he said we must learn to 'acutely sense and feel the movement of the breath within'. It would be wrong to introduce you to ratio breathing without pointing out that it potentially has this dimension. Of course, you will have already experienced some of this feeling in some of the earlier exercises; for example, when you asked your breath to create space forward of the heart, you felt your breath flowing in and down under your hands.

But now I have an exercise for you that focuses directly on feeling that movement, that flow of the breath.

EXERCISE 6.2: Pure Attention Nostril Sequencing. You will need to be in your CUSP, but won't need a clock or metronome this time. You may need to gently blow your nose to free your nostrils, one at a time.

Place your hands palms down on your thighs. Settle in with some easy, slow directional breaths. Breathe out fully and then turn your left palm up, focusing all your attention on your breath coming in through your left nostril. As that in-breath finishes, turn your palm down again and focus on the out-breath in the right nostril. When your breath is ready to turn round to an inhale, turn your right palm up and keep focused on your right nostril. When your breath is fully in, turn your palm down, throwing your attention back over to your left and to your breath flowing out through the left nostril. This makes one complete round. At first, you may need to ask someone to read you these instructions. Otherwise, continue for about five more rounds and then allow several free breaths before opening your eyes.

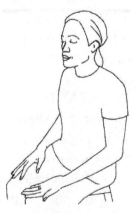

Figure 32. PANS: shown beginning with the left palm turned up ready to direct attention to the breath coming in through the left nostril

I call this exercise Pure Attention Nostril Sequencing or 'PANS'. It may have surprised you how the power of your attention shifted your breath from one nostril to the other!

Beginning Prāṇāyāma

One of the oldest and in some ways most comprehensive ancient texts on yoga breathing or Prāṇāyāma is the 500-year-old Haṭha Yoga Pradīpikā (pronounced 'HaT Ha Yoga Pra Deep Ik Ah') by Svātmārāma. I recommend the translation by Mohan & Mohan (2017).

The first exercise described by Svātmārāma is Nāḍī Śodhana (pronounced 'Nard Dee Showed Hanna'). It requires the Yogi to first close the right nostril and breathe in through the left. Then close the left nostril and breathe both out and back in again through the right nostril, followed by the reverse, out left, in left, with the right nostril closed. However, the value of Nāḍī Śodhana can only be realised if you 'acutely sense and feel the movement of the breath within' the nostrils. Simply going through the mechanics of opening and closing each nostril in the correct sequence will not create the desired effect, even if you work with ratio breathing. This is why I always teach PANS, the previous exercise, first so my students know what is the priority here.

We cannot think of starting Prāṇāyāma until we have learnt how to 'acutely sense and feel the movement of the breath within'. So, please repeat PANS, Exercise 6.2. That exercise, so long as you are breathing slowly and smoothly, is more Prāṇāyāma than simply opening and closing your nostrils. Once you have PANS established in terms of feeling what your breath is doing then you can, if you wish, start actually closing and opening your nostrils in sequence to augment the mindful practice you have already established. However, I suggest that for now you remain focused on the feeling of the breath in each nostril.

Nearly 20 years ago, I used to make visits to a student who was disabled by ME (myalgic encephalomyelitis), a condition that has much in common with long-Covid. She was barely able to practise any āsana, so I taught her breathwork up to the point you have now reached. On my next visit, I realised that through daily practice, she had become proficient in alternate nostril breathing. I asked what was responsible for her renewed motivation. Her reply was, 'Michael, while I'm doing this, I feel normal.'

Rousing or relaxing

I mentioned earlier that I started out practising my ratio breathing after work, partly as a way to relax. However, the exact ratio that will serve us best will depend on how we are feeling to begin with and what we plan to do afterwards. If you'll forgive me, I shall introduce two more Sanskrit terms, a pair of opposites called Brmhana and Langhana.

Brmhana means expanding or rousing; Langhana means contracting or calming. This pair of opposites was recognised centuries before the sympathetic and parasympathetic nervous systems were identified. If we are going to fit in some practice with the breath early in the day, we're more likely to need a Brmhana practice and in the evening, a Langhana practice will probably be more suitable.

Since most of what we've been looking at so far has had the objective of being relaxing and calming, the main change here is to talk about breathwork being rousing and energising. So far, we've concentrated on keeping the out-breath long, so it takes longer than the in-breath. We are ready, now, to work with the idea of the in- and out-breaths being of equal length in time.

EXERCISE 6.3: A rousing breath ratio. Repeat Exercise 6.1, but with both your inhale and your exhale the same length, up to 6 seconds and no pauses, i.e., a 6.0.6.0. ratio

We have also looked in detail at pausing with the breath out. Both longer exhale and pause afterwards, before breathing in, are found to be Langhana, provided they are not forced in any way.

EXERCISE 6.4: A more calming breath ratio. Repeat Exercise 6.1 or 6.2, now with a pause after your exhale. Try either a 3.0.6.3. or a 4.0.8.4 ratio. If in doubt, try the 3.0.6.3. ratio first.

Start, though, without the pause, taking 6 breaths to settle in. Then introduce the pause and take 6 more breaths. At all times, your breath needs to feel comfortable and for there NOT to be any strain.

McKeown (2021) says it's known from research (by Chapman et al, 2016) that going past the point of discomfort can adversely affect the very mind-body coordination which we are aiming to develop here.

Returning now to creating an early morning Brmhana effect, we need to keep the out-breath no longer than the in-breath and learn to pause before breathing out. And I'm going to throw in one more idea, to help you to work now on the length of your in-breath. See what this practice feels like:

EXERCISE 6.5: Putting a pause into your in-breath (Anuloma Krama). In your quiet place, assume your CUSP. With your hands on your heart as in Figure 33, ask your in-breath to create space forward of your heart. Stop, pause your in-breath there a moment. Then breathe in fully, expanding the lower ribs and so on down. Pause a moment with breath in. Then breathe out slowly, taking just long enough to equal the time you spent on inhale, pause and inhale. A metronome or similar may help at first. Repeat this breath sequence 5 more times, then remain inwardly focused on your breath to capture the effect.

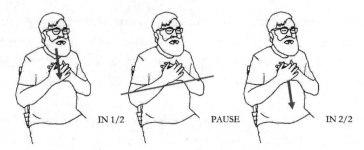

IN 1/2   PAUSE   IN 2/2

Figure 33. Anuloma Krama, half inhale to heart, pause for a
second or two, inhale more deeply. Exhale slowly

Krama means 'step' and Anuloma 'in the natural direction'. You
will have noticed how easy it is to use up too much of your
inhale capacity before you get to the first pause. Here we have
an exercise that encourages awareness of how you are inhaling,
of how much breath has come in and how quickly. So, with
practice, you and your breath will discover how to apportion
only half of your breath. Overall, your capacity to breathe in
more slowly will develop in this way. At the same time, you will
have a Brmhana practice to suit you for the mornings.

Let's look now at an exception to using Langhana in the
evening. Imagine that instead of arriving home after work, or
whatever, pleasantly tired, you are feeling stressed and dulled.
At these times, reach for your Brmhana practice. See if that will
lift you out of your enervated state, letting you fall back into
a more relaxed tiredness, more as if you'd been for a pleasant
long walk.

This is as far as I can take you, while still claiming to keep
things simple! However, if you wish to go further, there will be
other suggestions for you to try in the next chapter of this book.

EXERCISES SUMMARY CHAPTER 6:
6.1 Ratio Breathing
6.2 Pure Attention Nostril Sequencing (repeated)
6.3 A rousing breath ratio

6.4 A more calming breath ratio

6.5 Putting a pause into your in-breath

Step-by-step – 6

Completing the exercises in this chapter will have brought you closer to experiencing the traditional yoga breathwork, called prāṇāyāma, in a natural and progressive way. By now you've found and practised the sort of calming exercises I used to appreciate after a busy and sometimes pressured day at work. This more inward nature of your practice will help you to appreciate the subtle energy work introduced in the next chapter.

Chapter 7

Clear and Calm

Anyone who isn't lazy in the pursuit of Yoga, whether young, old, very old, ill or weak, attains success through practice.
Haṭha Yoga Pradīpikā, I, 64 trans. AG Mohan

Breathing is individual

While I've been working on this book, other books have come to my attention, especially James Nestor's 'Breathe' and 'The Breathing Cure' by Patrick McKeown, which I've already mentioned. As you will have seen, my book isn't, like Nestor's, a wide and fascinating exploration into the many things that can affect the way that we breathe and how that, in return, can affect our health.

My approach, as you've seen, is based on traditional yoga techniques, validated by scientific understanding. I see these two aspects being brought together by an evolutionary approach. In the roughly 1.8 million years that modern or near-modern humans have existed, their bodies will have adapted to breathe in a particular, optimal way. Such optimal breathing will have been observed and practised by the ancient yogis, since they also sought corresponding optimal health.

I'm not saying that optimal breathing is a rigid, one-size-fits-all. Firstly, we're all built a little differently. Secondly, small departures from optimum have little effect, so don't really matter. There is no need or justification to be exact. The individuality of the way each person breathes is one reason you won't find any cures in this book. My aim has been to help you find your way, ideally with the help of a teacher with whom you've developed some relationship, towards your personal optimal breathing.

Haṭha Yoga

What I've been sharing with you in this book is based on a branch of yoga called Haṭha (Hatt-ha). This yoga includes ways of working attentively with the body and the breath to create a state of physical and mental purity. In other branches of yoga that focus on meditation, knowledge, service or devotion, this purity isn't addressed in any detail; it may be taken for granted. Since the Haṭha Yoga was brought more to light by a handful of great Indian teachers in the mid-twentieth century, it has resumed its role of being an introductory form of yoga.

This makes Haṭha a branch of yoga which can help, these days, hundreds of millions of people who otherwise would have little if any interest in yoga. Its preparatory cleansing and clearing exercises can improve people's health in many ways. However, often this means that people rarely see beyond this initial attraction of yoga and often yoga is presented as mostly in the form of āsana (ahse-anna) i.e., postures, but with insufficient emphasis on breathwork.

Furthermore, the breathwork taught often depends heavily on Western sources, rather than being based on traditional Indian teachings. McKeown (2021, p22) says '...the Western psyche typically leans towards the idea that louder and bigger is better...the practice of taking noticeable, full breaths as often espoused in yoga is a technique that contradicts the original intention of yoga masters...' Quite so!

You may recall Svātmārāma's warning that working with your breath is like taming a tiger. The words he uses to describe the best approach mean 'softly, softly'. A little later, he says, 'One should gradually exhale the breath and as gradually inhale it.' (Adyar ed., Chapter 2, Verse 18). So much so that if your teacher were to hold a feather under your nose, it should hardly move!

Svātmārāma's rounds off his chapter on breathwork by describing the many benefits of Haṭha Yoga, including that of keeping you slim. This is when all he's described in terms of exercise has consisted of a handful of seated postures, such as Padmāsana (lotus pose) and advice on diet, but has mostly presented cleansing practices and ways of working with the breath. Apart from the bellows breath (Bhastrikā) Svātmārāma describes no strenuous breathing, yet he claims this yoga will keep you slim! How can this gentle, slow breathing have such an effect?

Your inner fire

The basis of Svātmārāma's claim that his Haṭha Yoga will make you slim is that it will brighten your inner fire. That's right, you have an inner fire! This inner fire, Svātmārāma would have told you, is located centrally in your body just below your diaphragm. Some of the exercises that I introduced earlier, such as exercises 4.7 and 5.3, will have had the action of brightening your inner fire. This will be especially true if your attention, as you breathe in, is on an impression of your breath passing through this region.

EXERCISE 7.1: Locating your inner fire. Sitting comfortably upright (CUSP), place your hand on a point between your breastbone and your navel. Close your eyes and breath in and down slowly and softly, past your heart and imagine your breath touching something internally, under your hands. It may feel like a gentle warmth. Please remember what I asked you at the beginning, to be patient and open-minded. After about 12 slow breaths, accept whatever you have experienced and open your eyes.

This inner fire that we all have is considered to have an important role in digestion, ensuring that food is fully 'cooked' in the sense that, once it reaches the intestines, it is fully broken down for assimilation. Krishnamacharya insisted that all food should, in this sense, be 'cooked' and it's also true that since our forebears mastered fire we have, as a species, become adapted to a largely cooked diet (Wrangham, 2009). Also, the nature and quantity of food is important, as insisted upon in the Haṭha Yoga Pradīpikā. Diet needs to be both moderate and pleasant, not too spicy or heavy, and alcohol and meat should be avoided or taken in moderation.

To maintain our inner fire, food and drink are not the only intakes to be regulated. Disturbing or depressing news items, especially if seen on TV, violent or exciting film or TV dramas, all tend to disturb our inner fires in one way or another. We don't need to isolate ourselves from the world, but rather to be a little more detached. Mostly, can't we learn about things the next day, sitting quietly with a newspaper, cup of tea, cat purring gently beside us...?

As regards breathwork, let us go on to develop and strengthen our relationship with our inner fire. As we feel the breath go in and down, the fire can brighten. As we slowly exhale, there can be a clearing feeling and effect. This isn't anything you need to be conscious of 24/7. I just want you to be aware that keeping your inner fire gently glowing is part of what I've termed optimal breathing – your personal optimal breathing!

Ujjāyī, or 'resistance breathing'

The breathing practices described in the Haṭha Yoga Pradīpikā can be categorised according to their effect on your inner fire. Some practices have a heating effect, by increasing the inner fire, some are cooling, by calming the fire, and some, including Nāḍīśodhana, are balanced, neither heating nor cooling. Ujjāyī (pronounced with 'oot' as in 'foot', oot-jar-yee) falls into the 'heating' category.

In my experience, Ujjāyī, like many practices, is best learnt in stages. Let's start with something with which I hope you'll be familiar. I call this 'misting the mirror'. First, have glass of warm water (ideally, warm cumin seed tea) to hand.

EXERCISE 7.2: Misting the Mirror. Assume your CUSP.

Part 1. Hold your hand in front of your mouth, which is slightly open. Imagine you have a mirror, or something else you wish to polish, in your hand. Breathe in through your nose. Breathe out through your mouth (for this exercise only!); breathe out softly into your hand, as you would to mist something held there by using condensation from your breath.

Probably, you'll have learnt as a child to make a soft sound in your throat as you do this. This sound in your throat is the basis of Ujjāyī. If you try again with your mouth almost closed, you will sound like the Star Wars character Darth Vader. What if you were to close your mouth next time you exhale?

Part 2. Breathe in through your nose and see if you can hear the same sound in your throat as your breath comes out through your nose. Repeat five more times, breathing in freely and out slowly, through your nose, but with this soft sound in your throat as you exhale. Take a few sips of warm water or clear tea, especially if this feels entirely new.

In my earlier chapters, I sought to help you slow your out-breath, for the sake of its calming effect on your system. Now you have a more sophisticated means to experience that, we can repeat some of the earlier exercises.

EXERCISE 7.3: Lengthening your exhale with Ujjāyī (Figure 34). This is a short sequence of movements taken over two breaths. In a relaxed standing position, breathe out slowly, placing your hands on your heart, ready to feel your breath lift them off, as in Exercise 4.3. With breath in and arms raised as in Figure 34, turn your breath around, asking for the soft Ujjāyī sound to appear. Let this help you lengthen your out-breath beyond the point when your hands touch either your knees or the chair. On the final second of your out-breath, relax into position. Then, breathing in and down, let your hands lead you into an upstretched, open posture. Again, as you turn your breath around, ask for the soft Ujjāyī sound to appear and smooth your out-breath as you return your hands to your heart. Repeat this sequence 5 times.

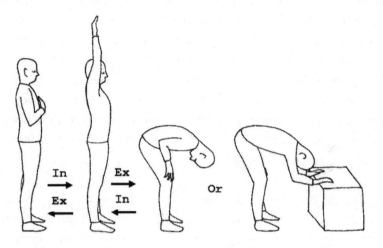

Figure 35. using Ujjāyī exhalation to ensure EX>MM

An optional additional bhāvana is to let your touch linger on your knees for a moment each time you start to breathe in, feeling as if you could touch the start of your in-breath to your hands/knees. Please keep your Ujjāyī soft; if you're new to this, it will be easier on your throat.

Sadly, I have sometimes been able to hear someone's Ujjāyī from several feet away. This is not the idea! I once heard one of Krishnamacharya's greatest students, BKS Iyengar, describe such a noisy Ujjāyī as 'egotistical'. I'm not sure I agree, but it's certainly not in keeping with the quiet subtlety we should expect from yoga breathing. Another benefit of Ujjāyī, or resistance breathing, is that pressure in the chest is kept up for longer, keeping airways open and allowing significantly more oxygen to be absorbed per breath. Pursed-lip exhalation, another form of resistance breathing, is recommended for COPD sufferers, so we can expect Ujjāyī exhalation to have similar benefits, while being more discreet, i.e., less obvious to onlookers.

Once you have established your Ujjāyī exhalation, there's an exercise you can do which combines a lot of the things you have both learnt and experienced to provide a firming and strengthening effect in your lower body. The short sequence of movements is the same, but your breath is employed differently. NB, this exercise is not advisable if you have any current irritation or inflammation in the abdominal area. Proceed with caution during the menstrual period or early in pregnancy. If you're not sure, replace Ujjāyī with the Ū sound from Chapter 2; if you can make a smooth, soft sound, this shows you are not straining and can use Ujjāyī.

EXERCISE 7.4: Moving between breaths (Figure 35). In a relaxed standing position, breathe out slowly with Ujjāyī, placing your hands on your heart as in Chapter 4, ready to feel your breath lift them off. Once your breath is in and your arms raised, breathe out fully with Ujjāyī, feeling your tummy lift in firmly. With your breath gently paused as in Chapter 3, take the forward bend 'on empty', relaxing into this position. Then, breathing in and down, let your hands lead you into the upstretched position. Again, as you turn your breath around, ask for the soft Ujjāyī sound to appear and smooth your out-breath as you keep your hands raised, shoulders relaxed. Pausing your breath, return your hands to your heart. Repeat 5 times.

Once you've got the feel of this exercise, you can think about setting some ratio breathing, as in Chapter 6. See if you can aim for 5 seconds each for inhale, exhale and pause, i.e., 5.0.5.5., either 5 or 10 times.

Another thing to try, if you've spent time sitting at a desk, is to get up, stretch your arms up and breathe out from your tummy.

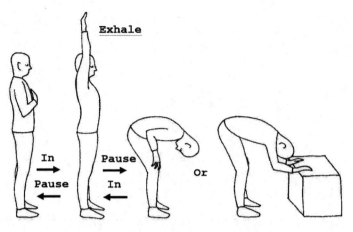

Figure 35. using Ujjāyī exhalation to ensure EX>MM

Ujjāyī and your inner fire

Although I've given the instruction to develop Ujjāyī on your out-breath, where it can be very helpful in keeping your breath long and smooth, the original intention, as described by Svātmārāma, was with Ujjāyī to be practised on the inhalation only, through both nostrils, with exhalation through alternate nostrils. But we're going to start with Ujjāyī first on exhalation and then on inhalation as well. This exercise will be another extension of the heart-first breath from Chapter 4. Have a glass of warm water (ideally, warm cumin tea) to hand.

EXERCISE 7.5: Developing an Ujjāyī inhalation. In a comfortable sitting (i.e., CUSP) position, close your eyes and gently point two fingers at the base of your throat, as in Figure 36. Keep breathing slowly and softly with Ujjāyī exhalation. Ask your breath what would happen if the sound could remain in the base of your throat, as your breath gently turns around and starts to come in. With patience, you will find that it can. Once you have established Ujjāyī sound on your inhalation, stay with it for up to 5 more breaths. Then sip some warm water or clear tea.

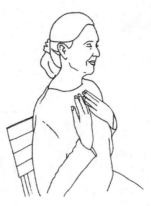

Figure 36. Using a hand Mudrā (gesture) to very gently encourage the appearance of Ujjāyī inhalation

Please repeat this exercise at least once a day, 3 or 4 times if you can. After a week or two, at least, move on to the next exercise (7.6). Think of enabling Ujjāyī inhalation as a milestone; it's a hallmark of proficiency for you and your breath. The name Ujjāyī is sometimes translated as 'victorious', but that success has only been reached thanks to a spirit of cooperation with your breath.

The term 'resistance breathing' was first used by researchers led by Dr Luciano Bernardi (Spicuzza et al, 2000) This form of breathing is identical to Ujjāyī; however, 'resistance breathing' is more descriptive for a scientific and medical readership. In 2004, Dr Bernardi and his co-workers provided a practical demonstration that slower breathing works for people climbing at high altitudes, improving the efficiency of respiration in the face of low oxygen availability (Bernardi, 2006).

Svātmārāma described Ujjāyī as 'sonorous from the throat to heart'. The idea is that, as you inhale, you imagine the sound accompanying your breath at least as far as your heart.

EXERCISE 7.6: Using Ujjāyī to feel your breath flowing forward of your heart. Assume your CUSP and come back for a moment to Exercise 4.2. You placed your hands comfortably over your heart as in Figure 19 (repeated here) and simply asked your breath, each time it came in, to create a little space forward of your heart. Please repeat this heart-first breathing now, using your new Ujjāyī inhalation to reinforce the subtle sensation we looked for in Exercise 4.2, that of the breath flowing in and down in front of your heart. Continue for up to twelve slow Ujjāyī breaths then with hands and arms relaxed quietly observe six more free breaths before slowly opening your eyes. You may wish to have a warm drink to moisten your throat. In time, you won't need it.

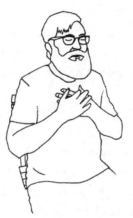

Figure 37. Bhāvana of asking the in-breath, with the help of Ujjāyī, to flow in a channel *forward* of the heart

Practise this daily until you are confident with it. Often, the sign we have reached this point is that we can do the exercise in 'autopilot' while the mind starts to wander. At that point, we'll have lost the feeling of breathfulness and it'll be time to move on to something new!

Ujjāyī inhalation increases suction in the chest, which will require both your diaphragm and your parasternals to work a little harder. Therefore, Ujjāyī can provide a gentle workout for your most important breathing muscles, as well as helping you once again to 'acutely sense and feel the movement of the breath within'.

Svātmārāma said that Ujjāyī can be practised 'standing or walking' (Chapter 2, verse 53). I don't use it quite this way, but Desikachar taught us to use it in our āsana practice to make the breath longer and smoother.

I mentioned earlier that Ujjāyī is considered to be a heating practice. This is especially true if we can combine it with a bhāvana, which here will be the idea of bringing your breath to what yogis call your fire centre. This is a subtle centre that feels like a source of motivational energy. Some writers have identified it with the solar plexus, but I hesitate to make the same connection. In my experience, I feel it to be somewhere internal between my breastbone and my navel. If, after trying the following exercise, this idea feels meaningful to you, just treat it as part of your inner experience.

EXERCISE 7.7: Directing Ujjāyī towards your inner fire. In your CUSP, repeat exercise 7.4, but with one hand over your fire centre. Add this visualisation, that as you direct your Ujjāyī inhalation towards your inner fire, that fire brightens and as you exhale, it returns to a soft glow. Continue with this breathing and bhāvana for 12 breaths, followed by 6 free, mindful breaths to integrate the experience.

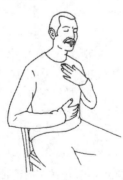

Figure 38. Sitting with one hand on the heart and the other on the fire centre

Potentially, this practice can be a way of clearing this centre, a place from which you can both feel some motivational energy and also speak with more conviction, as I shall now describe.

Voice-clearing

This I mean to describe both in the sense of clearing your voice and of using your voice in order to clear something. Let's re-cap a much earlier exercise:

EXERCISE 7.8: Using the Hrūm sound to feel an inner clearing. Assume the hands and knees or similar position that you used for Exercise 2.5. Repeat the movement, coordinated with your now long and smooth breath until you've got the hang of it again. When you have, start making a long HRŪM sound with your backwards movement. If that's a challenge to pronounce, start with RŪM or possibly BRŪM. I tell my students that an inner broom will sweep them clean. Repeat, putting some feeling into your voice.

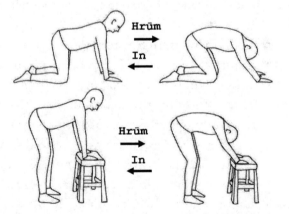

Figure 39. Kneeling or hands-on-a-chair HRŪM exhalation

When studying at the KYM in 2005, I asked about anger management. I was advised to chant a series of sounds associated with the sun, including HRŪM, because anger is located at the fire centre, which also has an association, naturally, with the sun. I found this chant had a very helpful clearing effect for my fire centre. So please feel free to repeat Exercise 7.7 when you need to clear out any feelings of frustration.

As hinted above, your fire centre is considered by yogis to be the source of strength for your voice, so if you keep your fire centre glowing clearly, your voice will carry more conviction. In the experience I related in Chapter 6 of dealing with an overpowering senior figure, it was my fire centre that supplied the calm but convincing tone to my voice.

This would complete my account of fire-centred breathing, were it not for the existence of a more powerful technique described by Svātmārāma, the Bellows Breath or Bhastrikā. The connection between a fire and a bellows is obvious! This deep and powerful technique is, however, not recommended for you at this stage, and Bhastrikā is a practice I intend to cover in a later volume. The Kundalini school of yoga teaches a lighter, but still effective, version which they call 'Breath of Fire'. If you are interested, please learn this directly under the guidance of one of their qualified teachers.

Cleansing practices

I'm going to introduce you to a couple of nasal cleansing exercises which yoga teachers will readily recognise. The first one I'd like you to think of as a form of 'rhythmic sniffing'. The aim is to repeatedly direct warm air into your nose from your fire centre. For this practice you will need to be able to hold your pelvic floor and lower abdomen gently but firmly inward for a minute or two, so please make sure you're going to be comfortable with this. Also, you're advised to work with an empty stomach, at least 2 hours after a meal and not be suffering any swelling or tenderness in the abdominal area.

EXERCISE 7.9: Rhythmic sniffing to clear the nose. Assume your CUSP. As in Figure 30, place one hand on your chest and the other over your fire centre. Create a firm, gentle tone in your pelvic/abdominal core. Breathe into your fire centre and then with a swift, light contraction from the same place, sniff your breath *outwards* and up into your head. Let your fire centre release, drawing your breath back in rapidly. Pause a moment and continue this rhythmic sniffing up to 11 more times, pausing for a moment after each in-breath to gather your attention. This is assuming that you and your breath feel comfortable. After about half a minute stop and pause your breath for as long as comfortable before inhaling again. If your approach is firm but not forceful, no pain or discomfort in the abdominal or pelvic area should result.

Including these pauses you will be starting at a breathing rate of 18-20 breaths per minute. If you feel that this rhythmic sniffing is going to be beneficial, a few weeks of daily practice will bring you to a point where you can complete 36 breaths in less than 30 seconds, without losing the rhythm or feeling any strain. You will also understand why the pelvic/abdominal core tone is so vital; without it, the force of your out-breath would be lost in a downward direction, which would be both unhelpful and potentially harmful.

Yoga teachers will recognise this rhythmic sniffing as a gentle version of Kapālabhāti (Cap-ah-lab-hearty), one of Svātmārāma's six forms of deep cleansing practices. Most of these are rather invasive, so Krishnamacharya taught only Kapālabhāti. This was consistent with his principle of using only air and fire for cleansing. 'Kapāla-bhāti' means 'head-cleansing' and its aim, as you have found, is to drive air rapidly through the nostrils. If you suffer from asthma, full Kapālabhāti is not recommended, please stay with the above lighter version.

Another cleansing practice commonly taught is Jala Neti. First you need to make up some warm isotonic saline solution, using 9 grams of salt per litre of filtered or previously boiled water. Then you pour it out of a special 'Neti' pot into one nostril and let it flow out of the other, working over a basin. Krishnamacharya did not favour this practice; however, I'm aware that many people do practise this form of nasal cleansing. So, if your teacher advises this, here are the things you need to bear in mind.

Firstly, you will need to learn the above light form of Kapālabhāti as an essential follow-up. Jala Neti can fill all your sinus cavities with saline solution, where it can remain for hours unless you clear it out with rhythmic sniffing. This will need to be done with your head still inclined over the basin, turning your head from one side to the other with each in-breath. About 18 breaths should suffice, followed by a pause in your breathing, while you wipe your nose. Repeat in an upright position, head still, holding a tissue to your nose.

Secondly, holding a cloth or tissue to your nose, rest your head below your heart, breathing freely. That should complete the clearing. Krishnamacharya would not have been aware of recent clinical and biochemical evidence (Ramalingam, 2019) for the role of saline solution in helping the cells lining your nose and throat to combat invading organisms. Surprisingly, they can use the chloride ions in saline to make hypochlorite ions (as in domestic bleach, but at much lower concentration) and target these at invaders. My conclusion has been that while Jala Neti should not be a daily practice, it's something useful to resort to when needed.

Mental clarity

This chapter would not be complete without mentioning the small, but in time significant, contributions that the practices in this and earlier chapters can contribute to your mental clarity. You will by now have observed this in yourself, and this greater calm and clarity will in time make an impression on those around you.

The Sanskrit word for mental clarity is viveka. The first man to bring yoga to the West in any strength was a Hindu monk whose guru, the legendary Ramakrishna, had most appropriately named him Vivekananda (clarity-bliss). Vivekananda didn't teach Haṭha Yoga; he taught the other branches of yoga that focus on meditation, knowledge, service or devotion. Haṭha Yoga, as I explained at the start of this chapter, is a foundational practice aimed at those of us who struggle with meditation and so on.

What these practices require is at least a small seed of mental clarity, stemming from your work with your breath. It is from this seed that the greater clarity developed through meditation can grow. Ultimately, we gain the insight to see ourselves as we really are.

We know our strengths and weaknesses, and know what causes us more or less suffering. We use the word viveka to describe this clarity...viveka means to see both sides, to be able to see what we are and what we are not...
Desikachar, p.90.

EXERCISES SUMMARY CHAPTER 7:
7.1 Locating your inner fire
7.2 Misting the mirror
7.3 Lengthening your exhale with Ujjāyī
7.4 Moving between breaths
7.5 Developing an Ujjāyī inhalation
7.6 Using Ujjāyī to feel your breath flowing forward of your heart
7.7 Directing Ujjāyī towards your inner fire
7.8 Using the Hrūm sound to feel an inner clearing
7.9 Rhythmic sniffing to clear the nose

Step-by-step – 7
Completing the exercises in this chapter will have given you all the tools to experience, if you wish, actual prāṇāyāma. You

are now able to approach breathwork with calm and confidence and to build on this calm and confidence by working with your breath. Everything you've learnt has now been brought together, all the basic things Mr Desikachar taught us, into a single, consistent whole and wholistic manner of working with your breath. Please congratulate yourself on reaching this level of sophistication! Your next step could take you beyond this book.

Chapter 8

Going Forward

This chapter contains no further exercises, but thoughts, ideas and links intended to help you going forward. We began with some basic ideas about breathing, such as breathing only through your nose, slowly, and feeling the movement in your abdomen in 'downflow' breathing. Then you learnt to be comfortable with pausing between breaths and developing a certain mindfulness which I'm calling 'breathfulness'. This gave you a platform from which to explore ways to helpfully focus in your chest on inhalation and to feel your breath working against gravity in a mild semi-inversion. Finally, you were ready to look at some of the more structured and subtle ways that yoga offers of working with the breath.

Where are we now?

While there are many more ways of working with your breath that I could share with you, these will have to wait for my next volume. You are now far more confident in your relationship with your breath. By this I mean not only that you have found within these pages some helpful exercises and have gained confidence about working with your breath, but also that you have by now more confidence IN your breath. That is, if your previous relationship with your breath was one of uncertainty, you are now more confident that whatever the situation, your breath will be either more ready to help you relax, or more able to support you if you feel challenged.

In these chapters, I've given you a toolbox of ideas and over forty exercises, so that you can now work with your breath in various ways. Not only will your breathing have improved, but you may have found relief from certain medical symptoms.

Also, your mood may have improved, including even the way that you feel about your body and your breath.

Please use this book, therefore, as a handbook of simple techniques, looking back through whenever you need some practice that is calming, rousing, relaxing or even uplifting. I've made it clear in the previous chapters that you are always to work within what is comfortable for you and your breath, your 'comfort zone', with no straining.

The directional breathing – downflow in from the top, outflow up from below – only needs to be observed while you are practising with your breath. Two of its aims are to open your upper body and firm your abdominal area. Most of your day, trust your breath to use the opportunities which your practice together has created. Then, whatever the need may be, it will work for you in the best way.

After a weekend retreat in Spring 2022 where I taught with my friend and colleague Liz Murtha, we received the following feedback about directional breathing:

When I went on the retreat, I was still suffering with extreme tiredness from Covid. The retreat was a really safe space in which to practice and explore my limitations. Naturally, I had energy dips over the weekend but, thanks to Michael and Liz's guidance, I came away with a good understanding of what I could do in my daily practice as well as things to avoid while I was recovering. In the days following, my energy levels really improved and within 2 weeks I felt much better. The key seemed to be the gentle approach to the asana, maintaining the balance between steadiness and ease, and keeping my focus on directional breathing – this breathing technique, in particular, has been very helpful. Thank you, Michael and Liz.

Jo.

Where to now?

Perhaps by now you have decided that the ideas and exercises that I've already shared with you are sufficient for your needs. You've found that you don't need to take your work with your breath any further, at least at present. In which case, the following words of advice take on an added importance.

More than one study has shown that people can gain considerably from working with their breath in a structured and motivated way over several weeks and months. They feel much better and, in many cases, can return to activities which they used to enjoy before their breathing or other health issues became a problem. However, in their now more active lives, their breathing exercises can get put to one side. For a while, this has no effect. Sadly, over a matter of weeks, the problems they previously overcame gradually return and they become dispirited.

If you're going to carry on working with your breath in order to hold off some problem, you must continue with whatever exercises, practised on a daily basis, have helped you the most. Daily, in this sense, means at least 5 times a week.

To go beyond what's in this book, or to find some personal support for your work from this book, you will need to find a suitable teacher, qualified to teach therapeutically and individually.

Finding a teacher

When I first became involved with yoga over 40 years ago, the idea of therapeutic yoga was in its infancy. Over the following 10 years, three people in the UK, the late Howard Kent, (Robin Munro www.yogatherapy.org) and Paul Harvey (www.yogastudies.org) began to introduce yoga therapy and to train people to teach yoga therapeutically, taking into account people's individual needs, rather than a one-size-fits-all approach to yoga teaching. I trained with Paul Harvey from 1987 to 1990.

Today, yoga therapy is one of the complementary healing disciplines recognised by the UK Complementary and Natural Healthcare Council (CNHC). The CNHC was set up with UK government support to protect the public by providing a voluntary register of complementary health practitioners. CNHC's register has been approved as an Accredited Register by the Professional Standards Authority for Health and Social Care, a body accountable to the UK Parliament.

For registered yoga therapists please search at:

https://www.cnhc.org.uk/yoga-therapy

Also, a professional association for yoga therapists (YTA) was being launched at the time of writing and will in future list yoga therapists trained with all the UK registered organisations:

https://www.yogatherapyassociation.org/

The register of those yoga therapy training organizations which train teachers to the high standards required to teach people individually and therapeutically is maintained by the British Council for Yoga Therapy (BCYT):

https://www.bcyt.org/member-organisations

This listing will include my parent organisation, The Society of Yoga Practitioners (TSYP). My colleagues in TSYP will be able to offer teaching, either in a small class or individually, which is closest in approach to what you have learnt in this book:

https://www.tsyp.yoga/find-a-yoga-teacher-near-you

The UK's largest yoga organisation, the British Wheel of Yoga (BWY), with which I trained from 1983 to 1986, and for which I ran teacher-training courses from 2007 to 2014, continues to train teachers to high standards. It's very likely that you'll be able to find a BWY-trained teacher in your area.

https://www.bwy.org.uk/find-a-yoga-class/

In the US, a number of my colleagues who trained with Mr Desikachar offer classes or individual lessons taught either by themselves or by their fully-trained students. These include:

The American Viniyoga Institute, led by Gary Kraftsow: https://viniyoga.com/directory/

Dr Amy Wheeler: https://amywheeler.com/about/yoga-therapy

The Breathing Project, led by Leslie Kaminoff and Amy Matthews:

https://breathingproject.com/

A wider register is held by the International Association of Yoga Therapists (IAYT):

https://www.iayt.org/search/custom.asp?id=4160

The following online search terms will help you find a teacher who can help you either to work through this book or go beyond it: Viniyoga; Desikachar; Patanjali; Classes near me

Finally, subject to availability, I can offer personal tuition wherever you are located, provided you have an internet connection and a device with Zoom software, a camera and a microphone:

https://twobirdsyoga.com

Becoming a teacher?

I hope that you've been so helped and inspired by this book that you want to learn how to share these teachings with others, by becoming an instructor or teacher yourself. If you are in the UK, I advise you to consult the BCYT, TSYP and BWY websites to find a suitable training course. These organisations will, however, be training you to teach yoga as a whole and not, as in these pages, a small selection of movements and postures focused on facilitating breathwork.

To help you to consider, my colleagues in TSYP can offer you a range of training courses, starting with Foundation Courses to take you from a basic appreciation of the potential of yoga up to a point where you can clearly decide whether or not to advance to teacher-training:

https://www.tsyp.yoga/training/foundation-courses/

If in the US, please try the links above. We also hope that there will be sufficient interest in our breathing methodology to excite research interest and, given that validation, lead to some focused training courses in key techniques for busy health professionals.

Are you a health worker?

What if you are already a healthcare professional seeking to widen your range of therapeutic options through teaching your patients therapeutic breathwork? Working through this book will, I trust, have convinced you of the effectiveness of the methods that I've been sharing, but you will know as much as I do, or better, that convincing patients and colleagues is one large step further.

You will also have seen that what I've introduced in these pages is, in one way or another, evidence based. The traditional understanding which we were given about natural relaxed breathing is consistent with modern research into respiratory physiology.

Social Prescribing is a potential new force in healthcare and Fox & Mason (2022) describe a 10-week evidence-based protocol, designed to promote self-care skills and bring about positive lifestyle change through yoga. This was trialled with the instigation and cooperation of the UK NHS West London Clinical Commissioning Group (CCG). The improvements in the health of participating patients, including their reduced needs for healthcare, paid for the ten weekly classes four times over. One driving force behind the integration of yoga into healthcare in the UK is patient empowerment:

Integrating health, social care, personalised care and social prescribing is partly an attempt to support patients to make the mental shift towards taking more responsibility for their health and wellbeing, and to give patients more control over their health.

Fox & Mason, p33

The breathwork incorporated by Fox and Mason in their Yoga4Health protocol will look very familiar to those of you who have worked through my exercises and may have shared them with colleagues and patients. I'm sure that, having done so, you will want to consult the growing body of scientific validation of the health benefits of yoga breathwork, some of which you will find referenced in the further reading which I've recommended.

Furthermore, please draw assurance from the fact that I've been drawing on the experience of Mr Desikachar and his co-workers at the KYM in Chennai, who have been applying and developing these methods with tens of thousands of students over 40 years.

Breathfulness for ICU workers?

If you are a highly-stressed health worker, a study (Klatt et al, 2015) conducted by researchers in Ohio may interest you. A cohort of highly-stressed ICU workers was provided with a simple, accessible mindfulness/breath awareness/yoga stretches program both in their workplace and on CD to practise at home. The researchers reported on the intervention (which was still ongoing) as follows: 'The intervention is delivered on site in the ICU, during work hours, with participants receiving time release to attend sessions. The intervention is well received with 97% retention rate. Work engagement and resiliency increase significantly in the intervention group, compared to the wait-list control group, while participant respiration rates decrease significantly pre-post in 6/8 of the weekly sessions.'

Looking at the participant ratings given to the activities in which they engaged, simple chest or abdomen breath awareness was rated by participants above meditation or stretching. I propose that a similar intervention using a selection of the exercises in this book would have similar or greater benefits in high-stress working environments.

Mental health

Working with your breath can improve not only your physical but also your mental health. This idea is very long standing in yoga; here is a key quotation from near the beginning of Svātmārāma's second chapter (my translation):

'What disturbs your breath will disturb your mind,
settle your breath and your mind will settle also.'

While it's not been my intention to assist you with any mental health issue, you may well have experienced some related benefits from the exercises in this book and wish to explore further. Also, working with your breath can bring to the surface suppressed emotions, such as grief or a feeling of loss or abandonment. If you are going to embark on a healing journey assisted by your breath, you are going to need someone suitably qualified and experienced to hold your hand, so to speak. Please look for support from a yoga therapist via one of the links above.

Breathfulness

Even if you are resolved to embark on a deeper healing journey, you will need to address some less-deep issues before you can proceed. This will require you to be mindful of your habitual responses to everyday issues. You will need some support in this, so I propose that you – and everyone else – can and should learn to be BREATHFUL.

About 15 years ago, Dr Jon Kabat-Zinn began to popularise the idea of mindfulness, taking it from one of his teachers, the Buddhist monk Thich Nath Hahn, although it has always been part of yoga (see Patañjali, Chapter 1, s.20, tr. Feuerstein, 1979). Kabat-Zinn (2017) defined mindfulness as 'awareness that arises through paying attention, on purpose, in the present moment, non-judgmentally.'

Kabat-Zinn continued by saying: 'And then I sometimes add, in the service of self-understanding and wisdom.'

We have an idea here of greater and more continuous self-awareness in whatever we are doing, saying or thinking.

As I hinted above, this mindfulness needs some ongoing support. Kabat-Zinn has, on occasion, brought up the idea, which I have also been promoting, of 'befriending your breath'. This is my reason for proposing the idea of 'breathfulness' or being 'breathful', to accompany that of mindfulness, or being mindful. Most of the exercises that I've given you in this book will help you into a state of greater mindfulness, through these moments of breathfulness, when everything seems to ride upon your breath.

About the Author

The author is a scientist who, for 35 years before he retired from a long career in physics, kept up first an interest in practising yoga, then in training to teach yoga and finally in training people to be yoga teachers, alongside a busy and at times world-leading role in a niche area of defence-related research. He has taught breathing at four World Yoga Festivals. In addition, he also managed to keep up his current interests, outside yoga, including travels with his wife, Linda, vegetable gardening and both reading and writing poetry.

***

From the Author: Thank you for purchasing *Breath for Health*. My sincere hope is that you derived as much pleasure from reading this book as I have in creating it. If you have a few moments, please feel free to add your review of the book to your favourite online site for feedback.

Author's contacts:
Website www.breath4health.yoga
Facebook: @Breath4Health
Instagram: @heartfirstbreath

Access is for news and answers to general questions and need for clarification. The author regrets he is unable to respond online to personal health enquiries.

References

Amann, M., (2012) 'Pulmonary system limitations to endurance exercise performance in humans', *Experimental physiology* Vol.97, no. 3 pp.311-318.

Benson, H., Beary, J.F., Carol, M.P., (1974) 'The Relaxation Response', *Psychiatry* Vol.37(1), pp.37-46.

Bernardi, L., Schneider, A., Pomidori, L. Paolucci, E. Cogo, A. (2006) 'Hypoxic ventilatory response in successful extreme altitude climbers', *European Respiratory Journal* Vol.27, pp.165-171.

Brown, R.P. & Gerbarg, P.L., (2012) 'The Healing Power of the Breath', Shambhala Books, Boulder, CO.

Chapman, E.B., Hansen-Honeycutt, J., Nasypany, A., Baker, R.T., May, J., (2016) 'A clinical guide to the assessment and treatment of breathing pattern disorders in the physically active: Part 1', *Int J Sports Phys Ther.* Vol.11(5), pp.803–809.

De Troyer, A., (1991) 'Inspiratory elevation of the ribs in the dog: primary role of the parasternals.', *J. Appl. Physiol.* Vol. 70, No.4, pp.1447-1455.

Desikachar, TKV (1992) Notes taken verbatim by the author at Gaunts House, Dorset, UK, 17 April.

Desikachar, TKV, (1999) 'The Heart of Yoga: Developing a Personal Practice', Inner Traditions, Rochester, VT.

Feuerstein, G. (1979) 'The Yoga Sūtra of Patañjali', Chapter 1, sūtra 20, Dawson, Folkestone, UK.

Fox, P.; Mason, H. (2022) 'Yoga on Prescription', Jessica Kingsley, London, UK

Gandevia, S.C., Hudson, A.L., Gorman, R.B., Butler, J.E., De Troyer, A., (2006) 'Spatial distribution of inspiratory drive to the para-sternal intercostal muscles in humans', *J Physiol*, Vol.573.1 pp.263–275.

Harvard Medical School, (2020) https://www.health.harvard. edu/mind-and-mood/relaxation-techniques-breath-control-helps-quell-errant-stress-response (accessed November 2020).

Hodges, P.W., Martin Eriksson, A.E., Shirley, D., Gandevia, S.C. (2005) 'Intra-abdominal pressure increases stiffness of the lumbar spine', *Journal of Biomechanics* Vol.38, no. 9, pp.1873-1880.

Holloway, E.A. West, R.J. (2007) 'Integrated breathing and relaxation training (the Papworth method) for adults with asthma in primary care: a randomised controlled trial', *Thorax*, Vol.62, pp.1039-1042.

Hutchinson, M.D., (2011) 'Headstand Day by Day' *BWY J. Spectrum*, Spring, pp.11-13

(No author cited) Imperial College Healthcare (2021). https:// www.imperial.nhs.uk/about-us/news/eno-breathe-national-roll-out (accessed January 2021).

Kabat-Zinn, J. (2017) 'Defining Mindfulness', https://www. mindful.org/jon-kabat-zinn-defining-mindfulness/ (accessed January 2022).

Kang, J-Y, Seo, D-K, Cho, J-C, Lee, B-K, (2018) 'Effectiveness of Breathing Exercises on Spinal Posture, Mobility and Stabilization in Patients with Lumbar Instability', *Korean Society of Physical Medicine* Vol.13, no. 3 pp.81-89.

Klatt, M., Steinberg, B., Duchemin, A.M., Mindfulness in Motion (MIM), (2015) 'An Onsite Mindfulness Based Intervention (MBI) for Chronically High Stress Work Environments to Increase Resiliency and Work Engagement', *J. Vis. Exp.* (101) pp.1-11.

Krishnamurti, J., (1964) 'Penguin Krishnamurti Reader', Penguin, London, UK. p94

Kuvalayānanda, Swami, (1966) 'Prāṇāyāma', Kaivalyadhama, Lonavla, India.

McCall, T., (2007) 'Yoga as Medicine, The yogic prescription for health and healing', (Bantam Books) New York, NY.

McKeown, P., (2004) 'Close Your Mouth', Buteyko Books, Loughwell, Moycullen, Co. Galway, RoI.

McKeown, P., (2021) 'The Breathing Cure', OxyAt Books, Loughwell, Moycullen, Co. Galway, RoI.

Mohan, A.G., Mohan, G., (2017) 'Haṭha Yoga Pradīpikā with notes from Krishnamacharya' Svastha Yoga Books, Chennai, India.

Ramalingam, S., Graham, C., Dove, J., Morrice, L., Sheikh, A., (2019) 'A pilot, open labelled, randomised controlled trial of hypertonic saline nasal irrigation and gargling for the common cold', *Nature Scientific Reports* Vol.9, pp.1015.

Sano, K., Kawashima, M., Ikeura, K. Arita, R., Tsubota, K., (2015) 'Abdominal Breathing Increases Tear Secretion in Healthy Women', *The Ocular Surface*, Vol.13, Issue 1, pp.82-87.

Schünemann H.J., Dorn J., Grant B.J., Winkelstein W Jr, Trevisan M., (2000) 'Pulmonary function is a long-term predictor of mortality in the general population: 29-year follow-up of the Buffalo Health Study.' *Chest.* Vol.118 No.3, pp.656-64.

Svātmārāma (15th c), Haṭha Yoga Pradīpikā, Adyar ed., 1972, Vasanta Press, Theosophical Society, Chennai.

(No author cited) University Hospital Southampton NHS Foundation Trust https://www.uhs.nhs.uk/Media/UHS-website-2019/Patientinformation/Respiratory/Breathing-pattern-disorders-patient-information.pdf (last accessed October 2022).

Spicuzza, L., Gabutti, A., Porta, C., Montano, N. Bernardi, L. (2000) 'Yoga and chemoreflex response to hypoxia and hypercapnia,' *The Lancet*, vol. 356, no. 9240, pp.1495–1496.

Wrangham, R., (2009) 'Catching Fire, how cooking made us human', Profile Books, London, UK.

Further Reading

For the general reader:

TKV Desikachar 'The Heart of Yoga: Developing a Personal Practice' (Inner Traditions) ISBN 978-0892817641

Patrick McKeown 'Close Your Mouth' (Buteyko Books) ISBN 978-0954599614

James Nestor 'Breath – The New Science of a Lost Art' Penguin ISBN 978-0241289129

Richard Wrangham, 'Catching Fire, how cooking made us human' (Profile Books) ISBN 978-1846682865

For the therapy professional:

John Douillard 'Body, Mind and Sport' (Three Rivers) ISBN 0-609-80789-7

Paul Fox and Heather Mason 'Yoga on Prescription' (Jessica Kingsley) ISBN 978-1787759756

Dr Timothy McCall 'Yoga as Medicine, The yogic prescription for health and healing' (Bantam Books) ISBN 978-0553384062 (see also his 2019 update at http://www.drmccall.com/uploads/2/2/6/5/22658464/yam_117conditions.pdf)

Patrick McKeown 'The Breathing Cure' (OxyAt Books) ISBN 978-909410268

Sat Bir Singh Khalsa, Lorenzo Cohen, Timothy McCall, Shirley Telles, editors. (2016) 'The Principles and Practice of Yoga in Healthcare', Handspring, Edinburgh, UK.

O-BOOKS

SPIRITUALITY

O is a symbol of the world, of oneness and unity; this eye
represents knowledge and insight. We publish titles on general
spirituality and living a spiritual life. We aim to inform and help
you on your own journey in this life.
If you have enjoyed this book, why not tell other readers by
posting a review on your preferred book site?

Recent bestsellers from O-Books are:

Heart of Tantric Sex
Diana Richardson
Revealing Eastern secrets of deep love and intimacy to Western
couples.
Paperback: 978-1-90381-637-0 ebook: 978-1-84694-637-0

Crystal Prescriptions
The A-Z guide to over 1,200 symptoms and their healing crystals
Judy Hall
The first in the popular series of eight books, this handy little
guide is packed as tight as a pill-bottle with crystal remedies for
ailments.
Paperback: 978-1-90504-740-6 ebook: 978-1-84694-629-5

Take Me To Truth
Undoing the Ego
Nouk Sanchez, Tomas Vieira
The best-selling step-by-step book on shedding the Ego, using the
teachings of *A Course In Miracles*.
Paperback: 978-1-84694-050-7 ebook: 978-1-84694-654-7

The 7 Myths about Love...Actually!
The Journey from your HEAD to the HEART of your SOUL
Mike George
Smashes all the myths about LOVE.
Paperback: 978-1-84694-288-4 ebook: 978-1-84694-682-0

The Holy Spirit's Interpretation of the New Testament
A Course in Understanding and Acceptance
Regina Dawn Akers
Following on from the strength of *A Course In Miracles*, NTI
teaches us how to experience the love and oneness of God.
Paperback: 978-1-84694-085-9 ebook: 978-1-78099-083-5

The Message of A Course In Miracles
A translation of the Text in plain language
Elizabeth A. Cronkhite
A translation of *A Course In Miracles* into plain, everyday
language for anyone seeking inner peace. The companion
volume, *Practicing A Course In Miracles*, offers practical lessons
and mentoring.
Paperback: 978-1-84694-319-5 ebook: 978-1-84694-642-4

Your Simple Path
Find Happiness in every step
Ian Tucker
A guide to helping us reconnect with what is really important in
our lives.
Paperback: 978-1-78279-349-6 ebook: 978-1-78279-348-9

365 Days of Wisdom
Daily Messages To Inspire You Through The Year
Dadi Janki
Daily messages which cool the mind, warm the heart and guide
you along your journey.
Paperback: 978-1-84694-863-3 ebook: 978-1-84694-864-0

Body of Wisdom
Women's Spiritual Power and How it Serves
Hilary Hart
Bringing together the dreams and experiences of women across
the world with today's most visionary spiritual teachers.
Paperback: 978-1-78099-696-7 ebook: 978-1-78099-695-0

Dying to Be Free
From Enforced Secrecy to Near Death to True Transformation
Hannah Robinson
After an unexpected accident and near-death experience, Hannah
Robinson found herself radically transforming her life, while a
remarkable new insight altered her relationship with her father, a
practising Catholic priest.
Paperback: 978-1-78535-254-6 ebook: 978-1-78535-255-3

The Ecology of the Soul
A Manual of Peace, Power and Personal Growth for Real People
in the Real World
Aidan Walker
Balance your own inner Ecology of the Soul to regain your
natural state of peace, power and wellbeing.
Paperback: 978-1-78279-850-7 ebook: 978-1-78279-849-1

Not I, Not other than I
The Life and Teachings of Russel Williams
Steve Taylor, Russel Williams
The miraculous life and inspiring teachings of one of the World's
greatest living Sages.
Paperback: 978-1-78279-729-6 ebook: 978-1-78279-728-9

On the Other Side of Love
A woman's unconventional journey towards wisdom
Muriel Maufroy
When life has lost all meaning, what do you do?
Paperback: 978-1-78535-281-2 ebook: 978-1-78535-282-9

Practicing A Course In Miracles
A translation of the Workbook in plain language, with
mentor's notes
Elizabeth A. Cronkhite
The practical second and third volumes of The Plain-Language
A Course In Miracles.
Paperback: 978-1-84694-403-1 ebook: 978-1-78099-072-9

Quantum Bliss

The Quantum Mechanics of Happiness, Abundance, and Health

George S. Mentz

Quantum Bliss is the breakthrough summary of success and spirituality secrets that customers have been waiting for.

Paperback: 978-1-78535-203-4 ebook: 978-1-78535-204-1

The Upside Down Mountain

Mags MacKean

A must-read for anyone weary of chasing success and happiness – one woman's inspirational journey swapping the uphill slog for the downhill slope.

Paperback: 978-1-78535-171-6 ebook: 978-1-78535-172-3

Your Personal Tuning Fork

The Endocrine System

Deborah Bates

Discover your body's health secret, the endocrine system, and 'twang' your way to sustainable health!

Paperback: 978-1-84694-503-8 ebook: 978-1-78099-697-4

Readers of ebooks can buy or view any of these bestsellers by clicking on the live link in the title. Most titles are published in paperback and as an ebook. Paperbacks are available in traditional bookshops. Both print and ebook formats are available online.

Find more titles and sign up to our readers' newsletter at http://www.johnhuntpublishing.com/mind-body-spirit

Follow us on Facebook at https://www.facebook.com/OBooks/ and Twitter at https://twitter.com/obooks